ADVANCED PRAISE

A rich and captivating personal exploration of growing old in an engaged, meaningful, and active way, The Seven Graces of Ageless Aging *weaves together Jason Elias's observations from his 40 years as a healer and acupuncturist with the lived experiences of clients and friends in older adulthood. Informative, enjoyable and full of thought-provoking quotes and useful resource links, this book offers many valuable insights on what elements may help promote and sustain a long, healthy, and joyful life into older age.*

—Nélida Quintero, Ph.D.

Executive Committee Member, NGO Committee on Aging/NY at the UN
Co-author with Sigal J. & Valente, E. (forthcoming), *Human Rights and Well-being of Older Persons: Challenges and Opportunities.*
Environmental Psychologist and Architect

Growing older is unavoidable but how we perceive this natural process depends greatly upon us. This book—based on Jason Elias's many years of experience and wisdom as a world-class healer—will inspire you to have a different perspective on the aging process that embraces the benefits of becoming an elder. A must read for everyone as they enter the golden years of their lives!

—Marc Grossman O.D., L.Ac

author of *Natural Eye Care: Your Guide To Better Vision and Healing*

When I first received the manuscript of this book, I said to myself: "Oh no! another task, another project, and I'm almost 80! I don't have time!" However, I read on with increasing amazement and delight, and found in Jason's Pathfinders, cultural creatives: scientists, artists, writers, now in their 80s and 90s – and over 100 –who kept their continuing enthusiasm for life and for creativity, even as by conventional accounts, it was all supposed to be over!

Jason's Pathfinders are not hapless "sinners waiting for redemption" at the end of their days, nor even monks hoping for samadhi/satori, though spiritual disciplines, seriously undertaken, permeate their lives. They are not waiting for anything! They are self-actualizing

for The Seven Graces of Ageless Aging

into the soul's next transformation! Read this book and Jason may help you, as he did me, not to fear death as the end of life, but its very flowering into a new becoming!

—Stephen Larsen, Ph.D.
author of *A Fire in the Mind: The Life of Joseph Campbell*,
the authorized biography

I'm sitting under a spreading maple, my dog at my side, and Jason Elias's marvelous Seven Graces in my lap. What a comfort! What a joy!

—Daniel M. Klein,
author of *Travels with Epicurus*

Those who have enjoyed Jason's earlier works like Kissing Joy as It Flies *are familiar with his storytelling mastery. Now, Jason wields his engaging and welcoming style to strengthen our radical acceptance, the courageous art of compassionately being alive. While the Seven Graces are illuminated through many interviews of individuals over 80, the lessons are important for everyone. They are ageless. Jason's findings are informed by empirical studies, spiritual philosophy, and, most importantly, delightful stories. Each chapter invites you to be fully alive in your own way, and to open the gate into your rich meadow of experience and explore with wonder.*

—Dr. Douglas Scherer, Ed.D., MBSR-QT, RYT200

The Seven Graces of Ageless Aging *is a call to live into old age fully, gracefully, with abundant health, passion, and joy. It also offers recipes for doing exactly that. Filled with stories of Pathfinders – ordinary people who offer inspiration through their extraordinary lives – the book also documents abundant research proving the efficacy of the author's recommendations for how to achieve an empowered old age. A must-read for anyone seeking the most out of life.*

—Ingrid Bacci Ph.D.
author of *The Art of Effortless Living*

Also by Jason Elias

Feminine Healing: A Woman's Guide to a Healthy Body, Mind, and Spirit

Chinese Medicine for Maximum Immunity: Understanding the Five Elemental Types for Health and Well-Being

The A to Z Guide to Healing Herbal Remedies

Kissing Joy As It Flies: A Journey in Search of Healing and Wholeness

THE SEVEN GRACES OF AGELESS AGING

how to die young
– as late in life
as possible

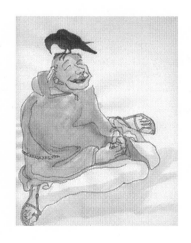

JASON ELIAS

CONTENTS

ACKNOWLEDGMENTS xi

A Note from the Author: Reflections on a New Normal xiii

PROLOGUE xvii

    My Own Reckoning with Aging xxii

    Facing Mortality – My Trip to Assisi xxiv

    Facing Mortality Again xxvii

    Turning to the Wise in Difficult Times xxx

The Pathfinders: Ageless Aging Personified xxxii

Introducing The Seven Graces of Ageless Aging 1

    Mind Over Matter 9

        Putting Placebo to the Test 10

FIRST GRACE:

    Rewriting the Script –

    reframing what it means to grow old 15

    Focusing:

     We Can Choose How To Think about Aging 25

    Choosing To Be Happy No Matter What 27

    Radical Acceptance 29

    Turning Back the Clock: A pivotal study 31

    Neuroplasticity: The Brain's Ability To Rewire Itself 35

    Reframing What It Means To Retire 37

    Cultivating the Seeds of the First Grace 39

    Online Resources for Rewriting the Script on Aging 42

SECOND GRACE:
>   Finding Your Tribe - honoring the importance
>   of healthy relationships   43
>   Choosing Connection over Tradition   52
>   Thriving Social Networks Enjoy Long
>   & Healthy Lives   57
>   Loneliness & the Brain   62
>   Cultivating the Seeds of the Second Grace   64
>   Online Resources for Finding Your Tribe   66

THIRD GRACE: Practicing Mindfulness   69
>   Spiritual Eldering   78
>   Transcending Stereotypes   79
>   Embracing Impermanence   83
>   Mindfulness & Stress   86
>   Meditation Practice as an Antidote to Stress   90
>   Mindfulness & Chronic Pain   91
>   Leaning into Discomfort   93
>   Cultivating the Seeds of the Third Grace   96
>   Online Resources for Practicing Mindfulness   99

FOURTH GRACE:
>   Awakening Joy through Simplicity & Humor   101
>   Decluttering Creates Simplicity   106
>   Simple Pleasure as the True Sustenance of Life   108
>   Laughter and Delight as the Best Medicines   110
>   Cultivating the Seeds of the Fourth Grace   115
>   Online Resources for Awakening Joy   116

FIFTH GRACE:
>   Pursuing Your Passion - clarifying a long-dreamed
>   vision or unrealized idea and practicing it   117
>   Creativity Late in Life   128
>   Suffering as the Alchemist's Flame   134
>   Cultivating the Seeds of the Fifth Grace   137
>   Online Resources for Pursuing Your Passion   139

SIXTH GRACE: Moving & Being Moved   141

     Moving as Essential to the Flow of Life   147

     Physical Activity Prolongs Life—Enjoy it!   149

         Keep Muscles & Immune Systems Young   153

         Just Walk   154

     Being Moved   155

     Cultivating the Seeds of the Sixth Grace   156

     Online Resources for Moving & Being Moved   158

SEVENTH GRACE:

Nurturing the Body, the Temple of the Divine   159

     The Ancient Chinese Model of Health   164

     The Basics of Chinese Medicine   167

         The Tao (Go with the flow!)   167

         Yin & Yang (Find/keep balance)   168

         Chi (Tapping into the life-force)   169

     Building Blocks of our Vital Energy   170

         Da chi (Wake up & smell the roses!)   171

         Gu chi (Feeding the body, feeding the soul)   172

         Shen chi (Getting/giving the love we need)   173

     Entering the Blue Zones   174

         Ecuador   174

         Japan   175

         Pakistan   177

     Inflammation: How It Works & How to Avoid It   178

         The Gut and Inflammation   179

         Food Sensitivity & Inflammation   180

     Moderation Is Still Key   181

     Staying Sexy at Any Age   182

     Cultivating the Seeds of the Seventh Grace   185

     Online Resources for Nurturing Your Body   188

EPILOGUE:

Living Unto Death & Facing Our Mortality   189

     Vipassana: Glimpsing the Beyond   193

     Embracing Mortality   198

     Living All of Life   201

     Assuaging Fear of Death: New Studies   202

ENDNOTES 205

Elderhood in Western Culture: Yesterday & Today 206
Egalitarianism Promotes Good Health & Longevity 208
Diving Deeper into Mind over Matter & Placebos 211

GENERAL ONLINE REFERENCES 215

RECOMMENDED READING 217

ABOUT THE AUTHOR 219

For more on our Pathfinders:

Iris Alster 71
Emelina Edwards............................. 162
Andrew Ferber................................. 73
Janet Hariton 21
Gillian Jagger 119
Daniel Klein...................................... 103
David Lewine 121
Betty MacDonald 48
Irving Milberg 3
Benedicta Nieves.............................. 45
Sarnie Ogus 143
Carolee Schneemann 17

ACKNOWLEDGMENTS

A book is like a wonderful multi-faceted quilt. Beautiful at a distance with its myriad of colors and design, but even more astounding when observed close-up. Each section becomes a tapestry unto itself. In writing this book, each individual's voice has woven richness and wisdom into this project's completion. It would take an entire book to properly thank those who wove this quilt, but I will note a few.

Catharine Clarke helped guide me from concept to completed project. Her rich editorial expertise and nurturance were essential. Lora Friedman's editorial skills and revisioning have made the book more accessible to a broader audience. Joyce Bellish brought our resource section to life.

I will forever be indebted to my Pathfinders, those individuals who have demonstrated and shared their joy in living a fulfilling life.

I encountered many obstacles—both from within and without—as we journeyed toward completion, ever-learning that going deeper into the darker spaces makes the light more profound. The consistent love and support of my wife and son pulled me through each time.

My dear friends and colleagues at Integral Health Apothecary, Marc Grossman, Lori Baczinski, and Mikio Kennedy have been steadfast in their support and make going to work/play a joy.

As I close these acknowledgements, I realize that the individual most responsible for my concept of aging gracefully is my teacher, mentor, friend, and father figure, Dr. Leon Hammer. I've known and studied with him for over 40 years and his support, vitality, and passion for life continue to this very moment. At 97 years of age, he recently completed a new book for practitioners of Chinese medicine. He took over a struggling acupuncture school in Florida, well into his eighties, and infused it with his passion and wisdom. It continues teaching and nourishing students to this day. I feel that his spirit fully embodies all of the Seven Graces. From the day we met I experienced him as an exceptionally wise being, yet always giving and humble. He continues to be a guiding light in my journey.

There are people in our lives who deeply touch us and are influential in making us who we are. I've learned that it is wise not to assume they know this. I have found that it is important to share your gratitude while they can receive it.

A Note from the Author:
Reflections on a New Normal

A near-final draft of this book was completed well over a year ago, but into the mothballs it went during a stressful time of selling our home of over 25 years and downsizing. The upheaval (and satisfaction) of "cleaning house" and clearing clutter took all of my focus, making it impossible to complete the manuscript.

When I again began working on this book in earnest after the first of the year, to rebirth it, so to speak, the COVID-19 virus all too soon began to wreak its havoc. Now, the world as we knew it has been turned upside down.

Sad as it is, it makes *The Seven Graces of Ageless Aging* even more relevant than when I originally started writing and compiling it. Not only are "we" elders facing our own mortality but our youth, too, must consider their own, as well as their parents' and grandparents'.

As we know, the COVID-19 virus does not discriminate between rich and poor, educated or uneducated, China, the United States, or the rest of the world (although the underprivileged are significantly more effected due to overcrowding and lack of resources). This virus has frozen our society and the world at large, and has brought the domestic and global economy into impending peril, creating a prospective abyss into which we are collectively peering.

I believe we can transform this abyss into a monumental opportunity. As I reread each of the Seven Graces, I realize that though they were written for the elders among us, they are relevant to *all* of us, young and old, as we communally confront the unknown.

Nonetheless, the pandemic amplifies the stressors elders more commonly face. We know we are much more likely to die from this virus than the younger population, and that social isolation can prevent us from getting the critical support we need. In addition to diligent handwashing, wearing masks in public, and socially distancing, we have many other tools and practices available to us to help prevent COVID-19 infection, such as:

- engaging the power of our minds to support our immune functioning;

- finding individual and constructive ways to center our energies and calm our spirit;

- taking this "opportunity" of free time to engage in a new passion or endeavor;

- remembering how movement and exercise keep us younger and more resilient, and

- how eating nourishing food and breathing clean air encourage good health and long life.

In general, we can transform our social isolation into opportunities for self-growth and for giving back by staying in touch with those who need our support.

My wish is that this book will inspire you, offer insights, and be a trustworthy companion during the no-doubt difficult days ahead.

JE/Autumn 2020

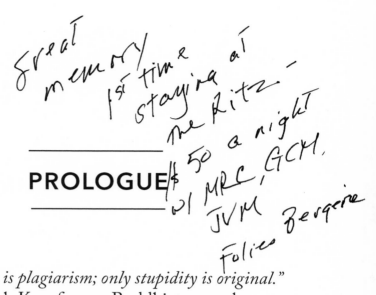

great memory 1st time staying at the Ritz - $50 a night w/ MRC, GCH, JVM Folies Bergère

---

PROLOGUE

"All wisdom is plagiarism; only stupidity is original."
– Hugh Kerr from a Buddhist proverb

"I have found that if you love life, life will love you back."
– Arthur Rubenstein, virtuoso pianist

_"Find a job you enjoy doing and you'll
never work a day in your life."_
– Mark Twain

"Old age ain't no place for sissies," the actress Bette Davis once said. She had a point. Thanks to modern medical advances, more of us are living to very old ages. Growing old can be a gift, considering the alternative, as has often been said, but living to a ripe old age can also be scary. There is no roadmap, but this book is intended as a primer of sorts, a compendium of personal observations, scientific studies, firsthand experiences, and feelings about "conscious aging that I call "ageless aging."

Most of the information in the pages that follow has come from a lifetime of study and from my experience, acquired over 50 years as a psychologist and practitioner of Traditional Chinese medicine, assisting hundreds of men and women as they have grappled with the physical, mental, emotional, and spiritual challenges of aging.

What is conscious aging? In my view, it means being present and aware as we go through the process of growing older and remaining as fully alive as possible, up until the moment we die. In this way, our age is ageless.

As living beings, none of us can avoid the reality of aging. Yes, we will die. Yes, our bodies will show inevitable signs of physical decline and we will lose some of the capacities we had when young. Regardless of how the aging process affects us, we can choose to live a vital, engaged life—until we take our last breath, or until our physical circumstances become intolerable (but that is the subject for another book).

In preparing to write *this* book, I interviewed more than a dozen individuals in their late seventies, eighties, and nineties, and one over one hundred. They are mentors, clients, and close friends. Each of these remarkable individuals, in his or her way, has refused to accept the timeworn script that equates old age with decrepitude. Instead, they have chosen to rewrite the script and embrace old age with dignity and grace. Listening carefully to their stories and insights inspired me and quieted my own fears about aging. They have become my Pathfinders, modern-day sages, who share their wisdom and experiences throughout this book.

When the interviews were completed and I took time to reflect upon the thoughts and attitudes about old age that my Pathfinders had shared with me, seven recurring themes emerged. I call them the **Seven Graces of Ageless Aging**. The Seven Graces are a distillation of the individual and collective wisdom of these courageous elders, whom I have had the privilege to know and love over many years, and who continue to enrich my life as I grapple with my own entry into conscious old age.

I am pleased to pass along their practical wisdom, and some insights of my own, to you in the hope that you will find them helpful in your own quest to attain a healthy and fulfilling old age. It's also my pleasure to share with you a broad array of research studies by respected scientists whose findings validate the intuitive wisdom about graceful, healthy aging that has been passed down from generation to generation, across cultures and continents.

Note: In an effort to ensure the continuity and flow of this narrative, the various studies will appear as Footnotes unless the study directly relates to a specific point. In that case it will appear within the narrative text. Additional Endnotes will appear at the back of the book.

Considering wisdom and old age, here is a good story to remember:

When Nasreddin was an old man, he sat in a teashop telling the story of his life to his friends.

"When I was young," he recalled, "I was filled with passion and the desire to enlighten everyone around

me. I would pray to Allah to give me the energy and devotion needed to change the world.

"Then when I reached middle age and realized I had changed no one, I prayed to Allah to give me the energy and devotion needed to change those close to me who, I believed, desperately needed my help.

"But now that I am older and wiser"—Nasreddin smiled and winked at his friends—"my prayer is much simpler, 'Allah,' I implore, 'please give me the energy and devotion needed to at least change myself.'"

"The years beyond 60, the years of our second maturity, may be evolution's greatest gift to humanity," author Jean Houston, director of the Foundation for Mind Research, reminds us.

We no longer need to compare ourselves to others, to fuss with our appearance, or worry about what others may think of us, all those thoughts that we have allowed to rule us, lay dormant in our mind-body. Now, we are free to explore, free to be ourselves. Social obligations mean much less, and we learn to care more for our own well-being than about meeting others' expectations. Aging calls us to look inward, to reflect upon our life experiences. We may release pent up energy from years of dutiful life and open ourselves to deeper awareness and spiritual practice. Current research also reveals that creativity often expands as we age. Freed from social constraints, we begin to trust our journey into the unknown.

This book stresses the value of reconsidering what it means to grow old while also reflecting on the true meaning of a life well lived. Such mindfulness encourages presence. When we remain present in the moment, acknowledging and appreciating even the simplest exchange or encounter, we enrich our life experience.

Many of my clients tell me that my office offers them a sanctuary where they can set down their burdens, and with my support they learn to trust their bodies to heal. Likewise, I imagine this book as a sort of sanctuary. It need not be read from cover to cover but rather dipped into, like a soothing bath for the spirit, whenever the moment calls.

My Own Reckoning with Aging

"Your vision will become clear only when you can look into your own heart. Who looks outside, dreams; who looks inside, awakens."
—C. G. Jung

Years ago, my dear friend Dr. Stephen Larsen, who wrote Joseph Campbell's authorized biography, agreed to read my memoir, *Kissing Joy As It Flies*, and to write its wonderful preface. Soon after the book's release, Dr. Larsen warned me, "Be careful, my friend,

I've known many people who have written memoirs and faced life-threatening situations, or even death, upon their completion."

His comment took me off guard. I thanked him for his insight but immediately buried his words, telling myself, "Not me! I'm only in my late sixties, still young. Having recently entered my seventies, I am content knowing that I have done with my life what I set out to do. I love my healing work as an acupuncturist and practitioner of Chinese Medicine. My patients appreciate me. I love my wife and son and they love me back. I've travelled the world. Nonetheless, my friend's strong words have lingered on the edge of my mind. Thankfully, so do Emerson's: "Life is not a destination, but a journey."

Until now, in my mind, it was always others who aged—not me! But, when my family and friends began to deal with serious illness and death, I suddenly felt vulnerable. Eventually, I had to confront the reality of both my wife's aging and my own. This ignited my curiosity and a desire to thoroughly explore the attributes, beliefs, and practices that promote long life with the invaluable help and inspiration of my Pathfinders.

Facing Mortality - My Trip to Assisi

In order to succeed, we must first believe that we can. I hope for nothing. I fear nothing. I am free. Since we cannot change reality, let us change the eyes, which see reality.

—**Nikos Kazantzakis**

Death is the wake-up call, the unavoidable mandate, that makes enlightenment possible, and helps our souls grow. This is why Plato, when asked on his deathbed for one final word of advice, he responded to his pupils, saying, "Practice dying."

—**Ram Dass**

As a kid in Brooklyn I liked to play in the neighborhood churchyard, where I marveled at a statue of St. Francis and his animal friends. (My father would drag me out, scolding "Francis is not Jewish!") While growing up, I read many books about St. Francis. I was especially fond of the masterpiece by Nikos Kazantzakis, *God's Pauper*, an imaginative retelling of the saint's life. In 1972, the film *Brother Son, Sister Moon*, a recounting of events in St. Francis's life, deeply resonated with me. Francis saw each living thing—whether a person, a bird, a tree, or a rock— as an object of God's love. He referred to each living creature as "sister" or "brother," as in Sister Moon and Brother Sun. His teaching reflected my priorities in the late 1960s and early 1970s when I, like many of my peers, rejected what I saw as the materialistic values of my parents' generation, and attempted to become unattached to possessions.

Fast-forward to the summer of 2016. My wife and I celebrated the publication of my memoir with a trip to Italy. We've always reveled in visiting sacred sites and decided to do a pilgrimage to the birthplace of St. Francis, in Assisi.

The saint's story continues to fascinate me. Sent out in the Crusades from Assisi to battle the Muslims, considered infidels by the Catholic Church, St. Francis came face to face with the enemy and saw that they were infused with the same divinity as his own. How could he kill a kindred spirit? Enlightened by this experience, Francis returned to Assisi, where he encountered hostility for what the community deemed his cowardice. He had come from a wealthy family of cloth merchants (the men in my family, too, had made a good living as clothing merchants), but, when Francis realized that their possessions were merely obstacles to the way of Christ, he boldly threw all the money and silk from his house into the street. When his father saw what he had done, he disowned Francis, banishing him from the family home.

From that moment on, Francis believed that his soul guided him to build a house for Christ. As he labored stone by stone, he begged for food so he could complete his task. In time, people saw the light that emanated from this humble man, the light of Christ, and many kindred souls helped him build his church and spread its love.

The night before our first day in Assisi I immersed myself in the Kazantzakis book. Soon I noticed that the dim light of our hotel room made it hard to focus and muttered to myself that I probably needed a new lens prescription.

When we got back to the States, I made an appointment with my friend and business partner, Marc Grossman, a holistic eye doctor. Marc found what he called "a macular hole" in my left eye. In response to my shocked reaction, he assured me that there was a surgical procedure to address my condition. A macular hole is a hole in the macular portion of the retina, which obscures the central vision. I would need surgery followed by a regimen of healing herbs and acupuncture.

When Marc asked if I remembered what I had been doing when I noticed the vision change, I told him that I had been reading the Kazantzakis book. He wondered what words I'd been reading, and I actually remembered: It was the story of St. Francis's mission to Africa, where he treated many people who had become blind from a particular blight that Francis, too, had experienced, and which caused him to lose his own vision. He proclaimed to the blind people, "In my blindness, I finally can see clearly."

Silence fell between Marc and me as we registered this synchronicity and its message. My unexpected health problem was a wake-up call. At nearly 70 years old, the time had come for me to confront and embrace the reality of growing older and to face my own mortality.

Having over a dozen clients in my practice who were thriving well into their eighties and nineties, most without any medications, I realized that not only could I learn from their vital longevity and therefore enter my own elderhood more gracefully, I could share their insights with others through my passion for writing about the healing arts. That "aha! moment" sparked the idea for this book.

Facing Mortality Again

"After a time of decay comes the turning point. The powerful light that has been banished returns. There is movement, but it is not brought about by force.... Everything comes of itself at the appointed time. This is the meaning of heaven and earth."

—The I Ching, Book of Changes

My wife and I, both then in our early seventies, were vibrant, healthy people with thriving careers in helping professions. We counted ourselves among the lucky ones in our circle of family and friends, for unlike so many, we had managed to avoid serious illness. But our luck had run out when my wife was diagnosed with cancer. We remained positive, but we knew that we'd reached a turning point.

In Chinese, the character for crisis also means opportunity. As Thomas Moore, the psychologist and sage, and others remind us: crisis can be a catalyst for embracing aging as the next phase of our life's journey, a time for deeper reflection, even a turn toward spiritual elderhood.

My wife and I began our approach to the daunting journey before us by drawing on the fruits of our lifelong meditative practices. We started our healing sessions in earnest, using imagery to send beams of light to attack the invading cells and shrink the tumors, and acupuncture to open the energy channels. My wife also began taking herbs to support her immune system, which we knew would be severely challenged by chemo.

We believed our ideal way forward would be to blend the best of Western medicine, targeted chemotherapy, with the gentler, nurturing strategies of the East.

My wife returned to work only a few weeks post-surgery, and, now, well over two years later, her health remains vital and she is truly thriving. More than ever, we appreciate each day as a gift.

I believe that our experiences of our own mortality offered us a life initiation. In the words of Thomas Moore: "You go through pain and worry, you reflect as you have never reflected before, and you come out the other end a renewed person. Over time, you take note of opportunities for initiation when they appear and respond openly and courageously. In this way your fate and destiny unfold, and you become who you are capable of being."[1]

Though this book has been brewing in me for some time, only now is the time ripe for it. I needed first to confront and embrace my own aging as well as my wife's brush with a life-threatening disease. I've come to appreciate how fully I love my life: my commitment to my beloved wife and son, and the myriad of nourishing relationships I enjoy with my clients and friends. I want to celebrate a glorious old age and share not only my story, but also those of the many elder role models I'm lucky to know who teach me, each and every day, how to live and how to age gracefully.

My years as a health care practitioner, many spent counseling and caring for the elderly, along with my

---

[1] Thomas Moore. *Ageless Soul: The Lifelong Journey Toward Meaning and Joy* (New York: St. Martin's Press, 2017) p. 121

lifelong love of "teaching stories," a devoted meditative practice, and a commitment to sharing my own elder wisdom, have inspired me to gather my thoughts on conscious aging and to organize them as The Seven Graces of Ageless Aging. Symbolically, the number seven represents the spiritual realm, as seven is not replicated in nature. Inspiration, I believe, comes from this source of our being, the universal energy that lives in all life forms. A grace represents an offering, a steppingstone, that each of us, at any age, may embody through conscious action.

Turning to the Wise in Difficult Times

"Do not seek to follow in the footsteps of the old, seek what they sought!"   **—Basho**

Even before the onslaught of the COVID-19 pandemic, we were living in the midst of pervasive political and social unrest. Unsettling issues already spanned the globe from climate change to the rise of authoritarian governments and the expansion of extremist ideologies. Now, with the onslaught of this virus still raging as I write in early May 2020, over 13,000 people have died in New York City alone, over one million worldwide. More than ever we need guidance to meet this peril, not only to survive it, but also to bring it into balance, renewing what has been lost and protecting what we must for future generations.

It's high time that we turned with respect to the elders among us, the wise ones, those with the long view, who have gathered the wisdom of their years and can share it. Conscious Aging asks us to shift our focus from retirement of the "no longer needed," to honor and embrace the wisdom in numbers among us. Perilous times are fragile times that require new strategies—where people are living to be older but not wiser, we must restore confidence in the aged, where our wisest resources have too long been neglected.

My wish is that this book may foster the re-awakening and re-emergence of the much-needed wisdom of the elders, wisdom that we desperately need to save ourselves and to save our planet from ruin.

May you, and those you love, age consciously, agelessly, with grace.

The Pathfinders: Ageless Aging Personified

"The idea is to die young as late in life as possible."
—Dr. Ashley Montagu

*"Light and colour, peace and hope, will keep painters'
company to the end of the day."*
—Sir Winston Churchill

I call the individuals I interviewed for this book
"Pathfinders" because their passion for living has paved
the way for ageless aging. Each of them embodies the
positive construct of aging gracefully. Our conversations
revealed these common threads of wisdom:

1. **They all reject the notion that aging means
   decrepitude and uselessness.** Rather, they
   believe that they have fully integrated the
   lessons they have learned throughout their
   lives as well as the gifts or burdens they
   experienced early in life. Now, in their
   later years, they feel less separate from, and
   more unified with, the universal life force.
   Some have remained active through creative
   pursuits such as writing, painting or sculpting,
   or have been generatively contributing to
   society through volunteer work. The desire to
   give back was repeatedly mentioned as a key
   impetus or motivation in life.

2. **Most expressed gratitude for a healthy body that could withstand the toil of many years.** This was particularly true for the creative types who, early in life had disregarded their bodies while fully engaged in their art. In old age, these individuals had come to realize that the body is our vehicle, the temple in which we live. They honor the wisdom that in the first half of life, the body serves us; in the second half of life, we must serve our bodies.

3. **All of our Pathfinders mentioned the importance of sustaining a sense of humor while growing old.** Many told jokes, and there was much laughter during our time together.

4. **Play keeps us in the present moment where life is always new.** "Pure play," one Pathfinder reminded me, "has intimations of the divine." He echoed the wisdom of Plato: "Man is made God's plaything, and that is the best part of him...Therefore every man and woman should live life accordingly, and play the noblest games...What, then, is the right way of living? Life must be lived as play."

In essence, as our Pathfinders show us, aging need not dictate dismal decline. When we debunk the negative preconceived notions of aging, we can even reverse the aging process. The studies cited in this book, along with the Pathfinders' collective, lived experience and my 50 years in the healing arts, offer solid guidelines, practical resources, and inspiration for those who want to learn how to follow Dr. Ashley Montagu's advice and "die young as late in life as possible."

INTRODUCING
THE SEVEN GRACES
OF AGELESS AGING

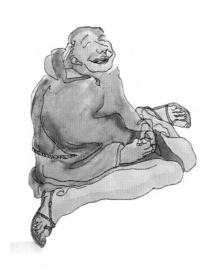

W e begin each chapter with an in-depth introduction to one of my role models, whom I call Pathfinders. Their indicated ages reflect their age at the time of my interview with them. Sadly, since that time some have passed on. Although all of our Pathfinders engender most if not all of the "seven graces," many exemplify one more strongly. Dr. Irving Milberg embraced all of them.

> *"Beautiful young people are accidents of nature, but beautiful old people are works of art!"*
> —**Eleanor Roosevelt**

IRVING MILBERG, M.D.
—— AGE 100 ——

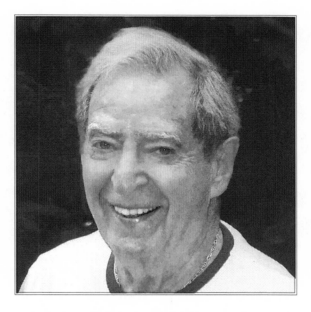

*When I first met **Irving Milberg**, he consulted me for chronic sinusitis. He had heard about me from a patient of mine, and since he embraced a natural way of living, like eating organic food and being an active tennis player, he was looking for a natural approach for his ailments.*

In chronological years, Irving was 83 at the time. When he walked into my office, I saw a sprite, wiry man with a youthful, bouncy step, exuding energy in his movements. His full voice radiated lightness, humor, and optimism.

He was a physician, trained in Dermatology as well as Psychiatry. At 70, he had retired from a successful Park

Avenue practice because "that was what people expected you to do," he shared.

He lasted only one year in retirement and opened a new practice in upstate New York. He said he loved his work too much—his patients and the thrill of solving puzzles. He believed in lifelong learning, keeping abreast of new developments in medical research. Irving was sharp as a tack, with an astounding memory and keen curiosity.

I had the good fortune to see him and treat him periodically for more than 16 years. He experienced only age-related afflictions like neuropathy and joint pain, none of which held him back and, in essence, he did not change until a year before he passed on at age 100. I interviewed him for this book when he was 99, and was not surprised that his zest for life, his relationships with his family and friends, as well as his keen interest in his patients, remained unchanged.

Dr. Milberg always emphasized the importance of eating a healthy diet, including abstaining from sugar and drinking lots of water. Irving also played tennis three times a week into his nineties.

We'd often spend the first fifteen minutes of each session telling jokes and complaining in playful ways about the state of the world!

The last year was more difficult for him: a fall and a bout of pneumonia had sent him to the hospital, and he had *to come to grips with taking down his shingle and moving, with his wife, three years his junior, closer to his son.*

I'm sure he would agree that he lived his life fully, happily, and without regrets, always buoyed by his thirst for knowledge, passion for his profession, and love for his tribe.

What was Irving's secret, and what might we learn from his long life? How can another person's personal path to graceful aging help us? At the end of the day, favorable genetics allow many people to live to a ripe old age, even with bad habits like smoking, eating poorly, and/or being secluded and sedentary, though these habits would lead us to expect otherwise. Reguardless of our genetics, role models like Irving have valuable lessons to teach us about not only living a long life but also a fulfilling one.

The associations we have with aging are often accompanied by anxiety and dread. Losing our mental acuity and physical prowess and the knowledge of our certain end fill many of us with such fear that we want to push any thoughts about it far from us. But exactly that denial can leave us more anxious and ultimately incapable of enjoying our last precious years. We often feel alone when encountering the process of aging. The younger generation can be empathic but is mostly unfazed. Other elders may be consumed by self-pity. At the end, we will go our path alone.

But listening to the stories of those who have managed, in their very individual ways, to find meaning and fulfillment in their lives to the end, often in spite of great adversities, can inspire us to find our own paths to graceful aging. It also connects us to a community of like-minded and spirited companions who seek enrichment rather than falling prey to the anxiety, fear, and loss in aging.

The Seven Graces of Ageless Aging synthesizes and simplifies the components of conscious aging into a primer for individuals who are concerned about their own aging process and for those caring for the elderly who seek an enlightened understanding of how all of us may approach aging more consciously and, gracefully. In short, these Seven Graces can serve as stepping-stones toward attaining emotional or spiritual wholeness as we age.

Elderhood can be a time of reckoning, a time to look inside, to wonder where we have been, and where we are *not* going. [2]

---

[2] The gerontologist Barry Barkan adeptly defines an elder as "… a person who is still growing, still a learner, still with potential and whose life continues to have within it promise for, and connection to, the future. An elder is still in pursuit of happiness, joy, and pleasure, and his or his birthright to these (pursuits) remains intact. Moreover, an elder is a person who deserves respect and honor and whose work it is to synthesize wisdom from long life experience and formulate this into a legacy for future generations."

In traditional societies, both male and female elders had specific roles and duties that balanced the losses associated with aging. They shared timeless teaching stories; they knew where to find medicinal plants and how to best use them. They guided the younger adults and became the caregivers and mentors for the tribe's children. Having experienced a whole lifetime, the community respected their wisdom, even if they were somehow debilitated. [3]

Today, professionals perform those duties once carried out by the elders. Looking about at the scores of nursing homes and assisted living facilities in our Western culture, we must ask ourselves: "Aren't these individuals, many of whom are cognitively alert, valuable to our society?" Of course, they are! It's heartening of late to see more and more elder communities being established that nourish these graces, but, as always, there's much more awareness to be raised.

The message of *The Seven Graces of Ageless Aging* is less about how to live a long life, and more about supporting vitality, being present, finding meaning and purpose, and sustaining a youthful heart—well into old age.

---

[3] Though Western culture has less regard for the wisdom of their elders, the anthropologist Joan Halifax believes that elders in traditional societies model developmental possibilities of old age, having become newly "innocent, clear-seeing, and compassionate."

The Seven Graces of Ageless Aging include:

1. **Rewriting the Script:** reframing what it means to grow old;

2. **Finding Your Tribe:** honoring the importance of good relationships;

3. **Practicing Mindfulness:** learning techniques that enable us to live in the moment (the eternal NOW);

4. **Awakening Joy through Simplicity and Humor:** living a simple, appreciative, and accepting life;

5. **Pursuing Your Passion:** clarifying a long-dreamed vision or unrealized idea and practicing it;

6. **Moving and Being Moved:** exercising sensibly on a regular basis to prevent stagnation and enhance mental, emotional and physical vigor, acuity, and creativity;

7. **Nurturing Your Body, the Temple of the Divine:** giving your body the essentials it needs to thrive (clean air, nourishing food, pure drinking water, and loving relationships).

Mind Over Matter

The beliefs our minds embrace have the power to establish foundational principles in our lives for both good and ill, either fostering health and longevity or ensuring disease and decrepitude. In fact, the power of the mind is the central theme of this book.

Each of the Seven Graces of Ageless Aging works with the power of our minds and our capacity to reflect upon and perhaps to reconsider our beliefs, even recast them, for our own good or that of others. We can shift our perspective on aging; we can detach from family patterns, commit to a mindfulness practice, and/or simplify our lives. We can look on the brighter, lighter side of life, letting go of overthinking. We can at last embrace a long-lost passion or come to believe that diet and exercise can truly make a difference in our lives.

The positive effects of the Seven Graces are amplified by our belief in their effectiveness.

Each human being carries the key to healing— physically, emotionally, mentally, and spiritually— within the incomparable power of the mind. The simple adage, "whatever we focus on gets bigger," applies here. When we harbor resentments, guilt, and blame, such feelings expand and cut us off from our inherent wellspring of creativity, compassion, empathy, and love—for ourselves and others. Negative patterns of thought and action reap what they sow. The power of the mind allows us to shift these patterns and, in fact, liberate our lives from negative thoughts and feelings.

The seeds of belief in the power of the mind to heal reach far back into ancient times. Long before the term "placebo" came to be scientifically studied and objectified, indigenous medicine men and women from multiple cultures adopted practices of deep and focused concentration to heal others. Today circles of intense prayer have been inexplicably successful at raising people from hospice beds; pilgrimages to spiritual places like Lourdes, Mecca, Jerusalem, and Sedona have been credited with miraculous healings.

When we embrace the power of the mind for good by changing a habit or changing our mind, we engage the brain's plasticity. Such newly adopted behavior, when consistent, rewires our neuropathways to better support our health and well-being.

Putting Placebo to the Test

Clinical trials in which subjects in a control group are given a placebo— a harmless treatment, such as a sugar pill or saline injection, in place of an experimental-drug treatment, indicate that many subjects get better after taking the placebo. This is known as "the placebo effect." (The Latin root of the word "placebo" is "I will please.")

While at an American Psychological Association (APA) conference many years ago, I attended a workshop entitled Modern Shamanism. After we were seated, the presenter walked behind a screen in the front of the room and announced that he was putting on his "shaman" costume. Soon he appeared wearing a white coat with a stethoscope hanging around his neck. He claimed that this attire would add 30% to his effectiveness.

I engage and employ the placebo principle daily in my acupuncture practice. The efficacy of acupuncture has supported good health for over 4,000 years, and herbal remedies for far longer. In other words, they work!   While administering the treatment, I intentionally speak in positive terms, emphasizing the client's innate ability to heal him- or her- self.

A client diagnosed with lung cancer once came to me after her doctor had pronounced, "Get your affairs in order; you have only three months to live." Devastated by the news, together we reframed her death sentence into just one possible outcome: She would survive! And indeed she did beat the cancer. (Her story is in my book *Chinese Medicine for Maximum Immunity*.) A negative pronouncement based on a medical diagnosis can potentially make a terrible nocebo imprint. (A nocebo is a detrimental health effect produced by psychological or psychosomatic factors such as negative expectations of treatment or prognosis.)

Maybe the person can expect to live for months or years, or perhaps even go through total remission, but there's no doubt that a verbalized sentence of certain death decreases one's remaining quality of life. In my view, such pronouncements amount to medical malpractice. Thousands of cases exist where people have gotten better due to a hopeful outlook, enjoying more of their lives than expected.

Dr. Ted Kaptchuk, a renowned scholar of East Asian medicine with whom I studied for my certification in Chinese herbal medicine, is currently a professor of medicine and global health and social medicine at Harvard Medical School. He specializes in the placebo effect.

Ted and his colleagues have investigated the neurobiology of the placebo effect as well as the psychological, cultural, sociological, and philosophical aspects of placebos. In one study, the researchers gave subjects drugs that could enhance or suppress the immune system, connecting each drug with a specific taste and smell. Upon discontinuing the actual drug, in Pavlovian style, they gave the subjects water flavored with an associated taste and smell and found that the placebo had the identical effect as the drug. In fact, the placebo produced the exact chemical reaction that the actual drug would have created.

Dr. Deepak Chopra, a well-known proponent of the mind-body connection, contends that a placebo "drug," usually a sugar pill of sorts, is as effective in 30 percent of patients—including those suffering from the side effects of chemotherapy—as an actual painkiller. Chopra also asserts that injections of sterile saline solutions have effectively reduced the size of tumors and in some cases led to remission of malignancies.[4]

Such a variety of positive responses to placebos indicate that our minds have the capacity to produce the appropriate biochemical responses needed for healing, based on the power of suggestion or belief.[5]

As we explore the Seven Graces, I invite you to be fully conscious of the power of your mind.

Note: See the Endnotes for more on "placebo."

---

[4] Deepak Chopra, M.D. *Ageless Body, Timeless Mind: The Quantum Alternative to Growing Old* (Three Rivers Press: New York, 1993, 1998) p. 18
[5] Ibid.

FIRST GRACE

Rewriting the Script -
Reframing
What It Means
To Grow Old

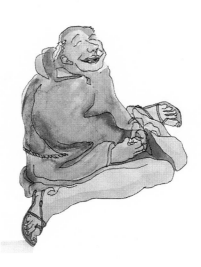

"The worst thing about life is death. That is why we all try to stave it off as long as possible. The first law of nature, we are taught, is that of self-preservation; but if you live in a society determined to eradicate you at a whimsical point, how can you observe that law?"
– Garson Kanin

"Your consciousness is your contribution to reality. What you perceive as real becomes real."
– Rumi

"Trying to hang on to youth, trying to hang on to what was great 20 years ago, throws you totally off. You've got to go with it and seek the abundance that's in the new thing. If you hang on to the old, you will not experience the new."
– Joseph Campbell

"In the province of the mind, what one believes to be true is true or becomes true, within certain limits to be found experientially and experimentally. These limits are further beliefs to be transcended. In the mind, there are no limits."
– John C. Lilly, M.D.

"Many seemingly unavoidable damages to our body can be reversed or ameliorated by the conscious application of the mind."
– Mihaly Csidazentmihalyi, Ph.D., author of *Flow: The Psychology of Optimal Experience*

CAROLEE SCHNEEMANN
——— AGE 80 ———

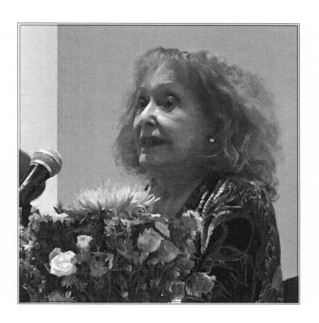

    Carolee Schneemann did it her way, from her youth
until the end. She did not accept her parents' demands when
she thought they were not what she needed. She broke many
societal rules and wrote her own script when it came to
the treatment of a grave illness. She succeeded every time.
Carolee lived her life with intelligence, determination, and
passion, according not to what others' thought best but by
what she loved, and she thought best.

Carolee ultimately succumbed to breast cancer in early 2020, keeping her diagnosis away from the public eye almost to the very end.

She was born in 1939 in Pennsylvania, her father, a physician, and her mother, a homemaker. When Carolee was a child her father encouraged her to accompany him on patient visits. Carolee was fascinated by the human body, which she learned much about through her father's anatomy books as well as her direct observations of bodily afflictions, blood, and gore. Her kind, loving grandmother, who had left home at a young age against parental wishes, was also a strong inspiration for her.

After her high school graduation, Carolee studied art but met fierce resistance from her parents. Her father threatened to send her to typing school. Carolee refused to give up her dream. Recognizing her talent, Bard College gave her a full scholarship, but her teachers warned her, because of her gender, not to be attached to the idea of a career in art. Later, Bard suspended her for a year because she had painted a nude self-portrait. She used this year off to attend classes at Columbia University where she met her future husband and partner of 12 years, avant-garde composer James Tenney. After Carolee received her MFA from the University of Illinois, she relocated to New York City with her husband and avidly joined the art scene. Her work became more and more diverse, using performance and videography alongside painting. She pushed against all taboos and explored sexuality and sensuality, often exhibiting her own nude body as a tool for self-expression.

She, and many artists that she inspired, rejected being objectified by men, and, in Carolee's words: "The very thing that has caused men to make us into objects, we will take ownership of."

Major recognition came late in her life. In 2015 the Museum der Moderne in Salzburg showed a retrospective of her art called "Kinetic Painting." In 2017, the show was a huge success at MOMA, and, in the same year, she received the Golden Lion Award for Lifetime Achievement from the Venice Biennale.

My personal connection with Carolee as a client and friend began over twenty years ago with her diagnosis of breast cancer. Her breast surgeon, a renowned physician, whom I highly respect, strongly recommended mastectomy and chemo to treat her cancer.

When Carolee came to me she had made up her mind to follow a path of natural treatment and to forgo, for the time being, any drastic measures. Her decision, she said, was based first on a strong intuition paired with her thorough research of the potential side effects of chemo compared to percentages of mortality.

She felt strongly that winning a favorable outcome with conservative medical approach versus a natural path *was not worth giving up the integrity of her body, which had become the central instrument of her art.*

Against all medical expectations, Carolee lived another 24 years.

These two precious quotes from Carolee offer words for aging gracefully:

"Be stubborn, persist, and trust yourself
on what you love."
"Keep sexually alive, eat kelp, and have a pet!"

JANET HARITON
——— AGE 82 ———

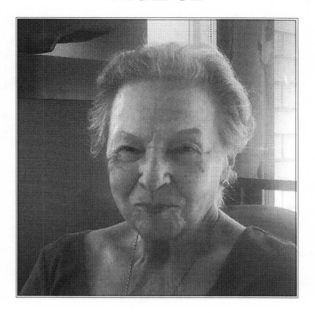

Janet Hariton doesn't only live her own passions, music and spirituality, she also is tenacious in her intent to wake up the people around her to their true calling.

Janet never doubted that she would live a long life since both her parents lived into their late nineties. It seems she never hesitated to follow her heart.

Born in Detroit just after the Great Depression she was sent away from her home to two aunts who were ministers in a spiritualist church in Michigan. There she witnessed spiritual rituals, healings, and communications with the dead. In her youth, she rejected those practices, but later realized that she felt a connection to this form of spirituality and was inspired by it.

From the time she was a little girl, Janet loved classical music. and had musical gifts. She has been playing the piano since the age of five. Her career was based on her gift for languages and she became a French attaché and later taught French in high schools. Later, through the friendship with a renowned pianist who became her voice teacher, she became involved in performing cabaret, which she loves with all her heart.

Married and divorced twice before finding the love of her life in her forties, she married a brilliant man 15 years her senior, a widower and father of three children— Janet struck gold. Her third marriage turned out to be the proverbial charm.

When her husband, an accountant and book author, turned 65 and retirement was discussed, Janet became nervous. She jokes that she was afraid that he would drive her crazy with his restlessness and intensity. So, she made it her mission to get him involved in some new occupation that would give him focus and a source of joy. Being highly intuitive, she enrolled him in a sculpting course. He resisted at first, since he had never done anything like this and didn't believe artistic expression was his forte. Yet at Janet's insistence he persisted, and a productive 30-year career of sculpting ensued. He felt the connection as soon as he started to use his hands. His last piece was finished at age 95. His art was shown in galleries on Fifth Avenue and some of his work can be found in private and corporate collections.

Janet had rewritten her husband's script from being a "numbers" guy to a prolific and successful artist who made a transition at age 65 that filled his later years with a deep connection to himself—and to life itself.

In her late seventies, Janet took classes and was ordained a minister in a spiritual church. She continues to sing cabaret, embracing her eighties with passion.

In the summer of 2020, Janet recovered from a prolonged bout of COVID-19. After three weeks of fevers, difficulty breathing, and extreme body aches and exhaustion, she is finally at home alone with her two cats. She shared that her belief that "she could" got her through along with the continual loving support of her tribes—her family and her spiritual community. Janet says she's ready now to give back.

Most of us believe the "script" about aging as handed down to us from family, clergy, teachers, doctors, and society at large. When we were young, we viewed our grandparents, parents, aunts and uncles as "old," even when they were only in their fifties or sixties. This no doubt created a deep imprint, a path that we assumed we would naturally follow. The script we internalized goes something like this: "I'm going to get old and feeble; my mind will go. When I talk, I'll repeat myself without knowing it. I'll lose control of my life." This bogus vision of a decrepit old age remains in our consciousness—and, if it remains unchallenged—can become our reality.

To become more conscious of the aging process, particularly our own, we must first consider our long-held beliefs about what aging is and is not. We would do well to adopt a "beginner's mind." This means not only learning the facts about aging but also realizing that our thoughts impact our feelings and our actions, resulting all too often in unnecessary outcomes. We can potentially decondition our programmed, automatic beliefs, and shift our thoughts into different feelings, actions, and results. As Deepak Chopra, the renowned physician and proponent of alternative medicine, notes, "We are the only creatures on earth who can change our biology by what we think and feel….Nothing holds more power over the body than the beliefs of the mind."

This reminds me of an experience I had as a very young man, when I worked as an aide in a psychiatric ward while studying toward my master's degree in psychology. My responsibilities included checking in on patients, taking blood pressures, providing limited psychotherapy, and reporting back to the psychiatrist and head nurse with my impressions.

One night, a young woman broke a vase and tried to cut herself. The entire front-desk staff ran to her aid to prevent her from slashing her wrists. I removed the glass from her hand, the doctors came, and I rejoined my colleagues at the front desk. Soon we discovered that while we'd been away from our posts, another patient had taken advantage of our absence and peeked at his chart. He saw that he'd been labeled "schizophrenic with chronic undifferentiated tendencies," a vague diagnosis that held little meaning. But the patient was unaware of this. After reading his diagnosis, he suddenly changed his behavior, acting bizarrely and hallucinating. Even when we explained to him that the label he'd read was only a designation used for insurance purposes, he started to believe that he was, in fact, schizophrenic, when in reality, he was not. In essence, he chose to become his diagnosis.

Focusing:
We Can *Choose* How To Think about Aging

"If you think you can, you can; And if you think you can't, you're right."

—Mary Kay Ash

When we were young, most of us baby boomers (individuals born between 1946 and 1964) rejected traditional assumptions about what old age should look like. We attempted, collectively, to rewrite the script and became known as a health-conscious, age-defying generation. Sadly, some of us have continued to chase the mirage of perpetual youth, indulging in excessive partying, plastic surgery, trendy fashion, fast cars, and the like. But the age-deniers have found no panacea. In fact, they're running so quickly away from aging that they are unaware of the beauty of their own naturally unfolding lives, and likely will miss the opportunity to truly prepare for old-old age.

But who can blame them? Societal attitudes toward aging and the aged, in general, all too often mock old people and portray them in film and television as undignified, ill-tempered, stubborn, mentally impaired, and just plain irrelevant. Becca Levy, Ph.D., a professor at the Yale University School of Public Health, conducted a study in 2002, which found that negative thoughts about aging could undermine health and produce damaging outcomes.

The longitudinal study was conducted across 20 years and involved multiple interviews with a large group of middle-aged individuals. Each person was asked whether or not they agreed with the statement,

"As you get older, you are less useful." Their views collectively revealed that one's beliefs about aging have more effect on one's lifespan than baseline good health considerations such as blood pressure, cholesterol level, smoking, or exercise. *The bottom line: Study participants who had positive perceptions of aging lived an average of 7.5 years longer than those with negative images of growing older.* [6]

I asked Pathfinder Dr. Irving Milberg, who was 95 at the time and still practicing medicine, how long he planned to continue seeing patients. He gave me a wry smile and said, "I keep rewriting the script." A similar message came from most of our Pathfinders, including multimedia artist Carolee Schneemann, who declared, "I refuse to age by society's rules. I make my own!"

Choosing To Be Happy No Matter What

New York Times reporter John Leland spent a year interviewing and getting to know six elders, age 85 and older for his book *Happiness Is a Choice You Make*. All were losing their strength; their skin slack, with many fading or prominent bruises. They didn't much like where they lived. In fact, none could say that tomorrow looked better than today. Nonetheless, they

---

[6] John Robbins, *Healthy at 100: The Scientifically Proven Secrets of the World's Healthiest and Longest-Lived People* (New York: Ballantine Books, 2006), xiv

all made the best of their circumstances, committed to living each day, no matter how hard, with gratitude. As one man named Fred said, "Happiness to me is what's happening now. Not in the next world…if you're not happy at the present time, then you're not happy. I have health problems, but they've been going on so long, they're secondary."

Psychotherapist Richard Carlson, an expert on happiness and stress reduction, coined the phrase, "Don't sweat the small stuff." (At some point, is it *all* small stuff?)

Like Fred from Leland's book above, Pathfinder Betty MacDonald, 86, believes we must let go of expectations and live in the present moment. She has long followed her creative spirit into psychodrama, sculpting, and dance and movement therapy. She told me once that one night while meditating, she had the striking awareness that her life was but a speck of dust floating in the universe, ordinary, yet one with it all. It was at that moment she understood that we have a choice to be happy, or not.

In his book, Leland cites a survey of people ages 74 to 104 conducted in the 1980s by Swedish sociologist Lars Tornstam. When asked how their values had changed since turning 50, nearly 75% of the respondents stated that they were much less interested in superficial social contacts; close to the same number said they delighted in their inner world, and over 80% said that material things mattered much less to them.

Radical Acceptance

"Flow with whatever may happen and let your mind be free. Stay centered by accepting whatever you are doing. This is the Ultimate."

—Chuang Tzu

Clinging to an old script or unchallenged belief about aging can bog us down with fear of death and despair, especially if we feel we haven't yet lived up to our potential or realized our dreams.

Depth psychologist James Hillman has observed, "The myth says that the roots of the soul are in the heavens, and the human grows downward into life. A little child enters the world as a stranger and brings a special gift into the world. The task of life is to "grow down into this world," not only, as so many of us believe, to grow up.

As we age, we grow psychologically and spiritually, seeking peace, wholeness, even transcendence. The time has come to accept our vulnerabilities and our losses, while recognizing our strengths and giving the gifts we've been given. This radical acceptance of our selves invites us to embrace even our *shadow*, as Jung called those parts of ourselves that we have buried, disowned, or banished to the unconscious. When we embrace all of our selves, we create space for new discoveries and new joys, turning first to what the world needs from us, and second to meeting our personal ambitions. When our wisdom guides us, we can guide others as mediators between the mundane and transcendent worlds.

Did you know?

When the Constitution was signed in 1776, a newborn in the United States could perhaps live to be 35. Today, thanks to dramatic medical advances and lifestyle changes, Americans have doubled that figure to 75. The National Institute of Aging projects that by the middle of the 21st century; men will be expected to live to 86 years old and women to 92.

In 1900, only 2.4 million Americans, or less than 4 percent of the population, were over 65. In 2010, the U.S. Census Bureau reported that 40.3 million Americans—13 percent of the population—had reached that milestone. By 2030, as the baby boomer generation ages, that figure is predicted to increase to 19 percent, or 46 million Americans. More than 80 percent of Americans alive today will likely live to be past 65.

Turning Back the Clock: A pivotal study that helped to launch the field of psychoneuroimmunology (PNI)[7]

"You're never too old to become younger."

–Mae West, actress

Ellen J. Langer, PhD, a professor of psychology at Harvard University and an expert on mindfulness, suggests that turning back the clock on aging is, in fact, possible. Her early work seeded her realization that making choices results in mindfulness. This awareness grounded her research in the distinct connection between mind and body. She came to believe that "we could change our physical health by changing our minds."

Langer stressed that society often expects older people to regress, to act like children, to give up their authority, their responsibility, and the essential control over their lives.

"Aging means change, but change does not mean decay."

To further ground her belief in fact, she and her students designed a study to explore what effect turning back the psychological clock could have on an

---

[7] Elinor J. Langer, *Counterclockwise: Mindful Health and the Power of Possibility* (Ballantine Books: New York, 2009) p. 156

individual's physical state of being. Though the actual year was 1979, they recreated the world of 1959 and asked subjects to live as though it were 20 years earlier.

They consulted physicians to clarify the biological markers of age, but found, to their amazement, that there were none. In effect, they found that scientists could not identify a person's age without knowing how long he or she had been alive.

In order to streamline the selection of participants for what would become known as the "counterclockwise study," the investigators established their own biological markers: weight, dexterity, flexibility, vision with and without eyeglasses—for each eye separately and together— and sensitivity to taste. They tested potential participants' intelligence and visual memory; took before-and-after photographs to document changes in physical appearance and asked each participant to complete a psychological self-evaluation test.

Participants responded to advertisements in local newspapers, which described the research as "a study on reminiscing, where men in their late seventies or early eighties would spend a week at a country retreat and talk about the past." Careful not to choose those who were ill, they selected sixteen participants, two groups of eight—an experimental group and a control group.

They turned an old monastery into a simulated world of 1959. The "experimental" group of men would live there for a week, going about their lives as though they were living in 1959. They were sent an information packet outlining the week's schedule, a floor plan of the retreat, and the location of their room. They were told not to bring any magazines, newspapers, books, or family pictures that were more recent than 1959, and to keep all conversations and discussions in the 1959 present. In addition, they were asked to write a brief autobiography, as if it was 1959, and to send the researchers photos of their younger selves, which were distributed to their fellow participants.

The control group attended a separate retreat a week later. They lived in the same 1959 surroundings but enjoyed activities and discussions about things that took place in 1959, rather than as if they were living in 1959, and also discussed present time. They wrote their bios in the past tense, shared photos of their current selves, and kept their minds focused on the fact that it was *not* 1959.

The researchers began to notice a change in behavior and attitude in both groups before the end of each of the two weeklong sessions. Upon retesting after the retreats, the researchers essentially found that, on most all counts, the participants seemed noticeably younger. The hearing and memory of all participants of both groups had improved. Each man gained on average three pounds with significant improvement in grip.

The experimental group improved more dramatically on joint flexibility, diminished arthritis in their fingers, and better dexterity than the control group. On intelligence tests, 63 percent of the experimental group improved their scores, compared to only 44 percent of the control group.

This study led Langer to firmly believe that it's less our physical limitations than how we see them, that is, our mindset, that actually determines how we heal and how we feel. This study opened the doors to this now thriving field of research, psychoneuroimmunology (PNI), which expands daily.

We can indeed reset the clock and grow younger!

Take Pathfinder Iris Alster, age 96 at the time of our interview. Iris believes in embracing opportunities. Her advice to all who have the good sense to heed it: "Say, yes! Then, you can wonder why!"

We cannot help but recognize the reality of aging. Yes, we will die. Yes, our bodies will become older and we'll lose some of the abilities we had when young. The good news is that, as individuals, we can affect how we will live and, to some extent, how we will die.

Try thinking of your body as your temple, your mind as your universe, and your heart as your gold.

Neuroplasticity:
The Brain's Ability To Rewire Itself

The essence of quantum physics reveals that when we're open to learning and embracing new beliefs, that the neurons in the brain have the capacity to add new connections, forge new pathways through the cortex, and even take on new roles. The brain's ability to rewire itself is called neuroplasticity. Brain-generating neurons allow us to change our thinking, our feelings, and our patterned beliefs.

Intention and its companion, attention, offer active tools for shifting long-held beliefs. We can make once-automatic choices conscious. Why not take charge of your brain and tell it that you *intend* to live a vigorous, healthy life, well into old age? Giving dedicated attention to this intention can precipitate a shift from the old script to the new.

Pathfinder Dr. Andrew Ferber, 86, psychiatrist, spiritual teacher, and former professor of family therapy at the Albert Einstein College of Medicine in New York City, who is also known as Bodhicitta, shared this with me:

"I believe each of us has a deep, inner wisdom, an inner guidance. All of my experiences begin with that belief. When I was in medical school, I somehow knew that what they were teaching me remained in a box—not a bad box, a good one—but a limited one. I knew that the truth was much bigger that what I was being taught. I've always been naturally drawn to holistic medicine, anti-aging, and relying on myself in body and mind. I say, 'Stop believing that you're old, do what feels natural to you.'"

I recently reunited, after nearly 30 years, with Pathfinder Sarnie Ogus, one of my trainers in the Alexander Technique. Sarnie was age 93 at this writing and still youthful in both her energy and demeanor.

When I asked Sarnie if she'd had a role model in her youth who represented personal accountability for her, she smiled ruefully and said, "I guess that would be my sister. She was 15 years my senior, and I think she was committed to the decrepitude of aging. I learned fast, from her example, what I didn't want to be."

Just before we ended our time together, Sarnie shared these wise and simple words, "When your mind makes a contract that your body can't fulfill, you're old—until you make a new contract."

Some of us learn how *not* to be by watching others; others rely on intuition or inner guidance, particularly if they value their inner life and practice some form of awareness.

Reframing What It Means To Retire

Our youth-oriented culture tells us that 65 is the new 55, and that retirement can open doorways to creativity and freedom. But, when a person is forced to retire after spending many years in the workplace, life can begin to lose its meaning. Depression can set in.

The very words "retire" or "retirement" perpetuate the myth that old age is an unproductive time in life and imprints the belief that people in their later years should simply sit back or indulge in a recreational activity like golf. (Ironically, the word recreate or "re-create," essentially means, "to create anew.")

Gustav Eckstein, a medical doctor, scientist, teacher, and philosopher, who, in 1935, studied with Ivan Pavlov, a pioneer in the field of conditioned reflexes, said this: "The trouble with mandatory retirement is: If you tell a man he's going to be retired on his 65th birthday, it's much the same as telling a man sitting on death row that he's going to be executed on such and such a date; he begins to fade. He's conditioned—how well Pavlov understood this....(The man's) been told repeatedly that 65 equals uselessness. If we're told something over and over again, no matter how nonsensical, we believe it." [8]

It's no wonder that the suicide rate for retired men is 12 times higher than for those who are employed. Society, the government, and the law tell them they are finished. A concept tinged with uselessness, as Dr. Eckstein noted, retirement essentially put the final nails in my own father's coffin; he felt sentenced to being "over the hill" with nothing worthwhile left to give.

In India, when an individual reaches 50 or 60 years old, he or she enters the time of *sanyas*, when worldly concerns have been fulfilled, and the time has come to give back to his or her community, growing older and wiser naturally. Their focus turns to spirit, the eternal light within. Death becomes a celebration, a return to the light. An attitude and awareness of such an unfolding destination in later life reframes the meaning of retirement.

In Native American culture, the grandmothers, the wisest among the tribe, call the postmenopausal women to the Grandmother Lodge. (The elder men have their own council.) These grandmothers carry the great visions not only for the family—the work

---

[8] Ibid. p. 91

of the menstrual women of the Moon Lodge— but also for the entire tribe. Here there is no "retirement." The purpose of the Grandmother Lodge is to offer the postmenopausal women retreat from daily duties so that they can be receptive to their visions for the benefit of the entire community.

Through all of the Blue Zones, communities, which can expect many to reach into the 100s, retirement doesn't exist. These elders continue to farm, fish, and follow their regular routines, until it becomes time to better use their skills by caring for and passing their wisdom to the children of their communities.

Whether we embrace our retirement as open time for creative pursuits after a lifetime of dutiful daily work or choose to continue our life work for the rest of our days, our elder years offer each of us the possibility of both embracing our heart's desires and giving back to a world, a life, that has given us so much.

Cultivating the Seeds of the First Grace: Rewriting the script

"When I let go of what I am, I become what I might be."
—Lao Tzu

The seed carries the essence of a plant, much like the spark of a new idea before it becomes a reality.

When we plant a seed, whether in our literal garden or in our garden of new ideas, we must nourish that seed. To reframe the meaning of aging in your own life and encourage ageless aging, here are a few suggestions to guide your shift:

1. **Pay attention to your reactive thoughts**, which all too often can be negative in our current divisive political environment. Reverse them. Let the positive thoughts stick and the negative ones roll away.

2. **Pay attention to your words and catch yourself when your mind says, "I can't do that!"** Recall a recent time when you confronted the "I can't" with "I can, and I did!" Remember that.

3. **Find small things you can do to make a difference.** No one is useless. For example, a friend started a business with the simple idea that we can "change the world, one bag at a time!" She began a company called Eco-bags, and indeed makes a big difference to the world, and a good living as well, by supplying reusable, sustainable shopping bags.

4. **Ask yourself if your old, habitual story is true?** I've always said that I'm not lucky when it comes to money. My wife recently pointed

out that this belief inhibits attracting material abundance. She suggests changing the script to "There's nothing wrong with making money." Don't sell yourself short; say, "I'm worth it!"

5. **Use positive affirmations** such as Emily Coue's "Every day in every way, I'm getting better and better." Or, "Aging is reversible." Remember, neuroplasticity gives us the choice to change our neural pathways by dropping worn-out, conditioned thoughts and beliefs. Find affirmations that resonate with you. Write them down on Post-it notes and place them where you can see them: on your refrigerator door, near your computer, by your bedside, or on your bathroom mirror.

6. **Look for elders with whom you resonate,** who represent a new model of aging. Affirm that, "I too, can stay young, very late into life." Don't focus on the negative stereotypes of aging that we see on our screens, modeled by so many. We have the power to affirm the positive and "delete" the negative.

7. **Learn to observe your thoughts without judging.** If you hear yourself saying things that perpetuate the myth of aging and decrepitude, re-focus your thought.

Online Resources
for Rewriting the Script on Aging

Aging with style:

https://www.bbc.com/culture/article/20141110-growing-old-disgracefully

This is what growing old really looks like:

https://www.nextavenue.org/slideshow/pictures-growing-old/#slide13

What's being done to reframe aging?

https://www.asaging.org/reframing-aging

Reframing Aging Tool Kit:

https://www.johnahartford.org/events/view/reframing-aging-issue-brief-released/

Center for Conscious Eldering:

https://www.centerforconsciouseldering.com

SECOND GRACE

Finding Your Tribe -
honoring the importance
of healthy relationships

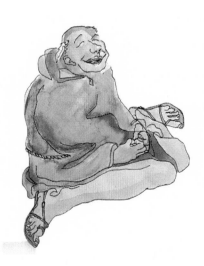

"The heart that loves is always young."
—Greek proverb

"Everyone on earth belongs to a spirit clan. The problem is that you have to find it."

—Lynn Andrews, *Flight of the Seventh Moon*

"Let there be no purpose in friendship save the deepening of spirit."
—Kahil Gibran

"My tribe comes to me at each phase of my life."
—Pathfinder Benedicta Nieves

"I have the most amazing friends and community! It's beyond Ananda (bliss)."
—Pathfinder David Lewine

"Margaret Mead defined an ideal community as one that has a place for every human gift."
—Mary Piper

BENEDICTA NIEVES
── AGE 88 ──

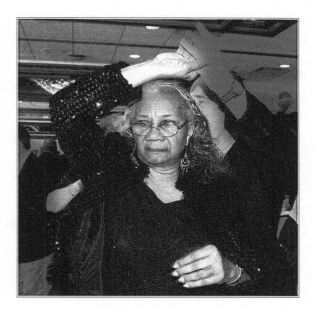

Benedicta Nieves always had a very strong sense of belonging. Her self-possessed identity came from belonging to the "tribe" of her original family. But, over the years, she added a variety of new and diverse groups of people with whom she also felt strong connections. This helped her through many hardships and, to this day, is essential to her happiness.

Benedicta was born in Puerto Rico into a large family in which music and dance were an essential part of daily life. Everyone who could worked hard, mostly manual labor, however, in every minute of down-time music permeated the home and neighborhood. Young children, elders, and everyone in between played an instrument. Elders were highly respected in Benedicta's community.

Her father died young, and when Benedicta was only 12, she and her mother moved to the United States to increase their income and help their family back in Puerto Rico. Her mother believed anything was possible in America, and so did Benedicta, who helped out as a seamstress. They lived in Brooklyn in a mostly Puerto Rican neighborhood.

Benedicta's mother supported her little girl's passion for dance and enrolled her in ballet classes. Dance became a lifelong passion for Benedicta.

Although she was a good student, Benedicta's dream of becoming a medical doctor was not to be. Her parents did not have the resources to provide her with a first-class education, but she did go to college after high school. Benedicta got married as an undergraduate and had three children at a young age. Her husband supported her, and after graduation she attended a master's program in Albany in bilingual education.

Benedicta's beloved husband died young and tragically, shortly after, her youngest child, a nine-year-old daughter, died of leukemia. She was devastated but teaching kept her going. She accepted a job as a Spanish teacher in Beacon, New York, which eventually led to a directorship of the Bi-lingual Department of the Hyde Park school system. Teaching became the path to a new tribe. Her colleagues and students became a new family and a new source of identity. She talks about her students with great affection. Sharing knowledge and the wish to better herself made her happy.

When her second child died in his mid-fifties, Benedicta fell into a deep crisis. She questioned why she should live while the three closest to her had died. In her depression, it came to her how music had bonded her to her family of origin and that it had always held healing power for her. Through music she found her way back and through dance she embraced being alive again. Dancing, above all, she says "fills my soul," but yoga, tai chi and Zumba, as well as her new-found, deep love of meditation have helped her let go of negative thoughts.

Today, at 88, Benedicta teaches language courses and dance to elders at a senior citizens center in Poughkeepsie, New York. She continues to take courses there and currently studies German and takes guitar lessons. Sharing her passions with her new and old tribes, and, last but not least, her son and grandchildren, keep her young and vibrant.

BETTY MacDONALD
——— AGE 86 ———

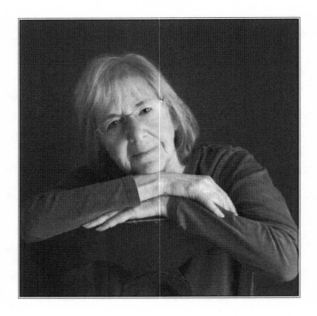

Betty MacDonald has been a patient of mine for 25 years. I am her "doctor for well-being and prevention." She lives by herself in a small house surrounded by the magic of nature. Enthusiastically and religiously, she practices Pilates and yoga and only eats organic products from a local food coop. Very recently Betty even took up tap dancing. But her primary passion is her engagement with her children, 11 grandchildren, and a vast network of close friends, her "tribe."

Betty told me during our interview for this book that finding a true feeling of belonging and connection did not come easy for her. In the search for her "tribe" she took circuitous routes.

Betty was born in Richmond, Virginia, to Eastern European immigrants, who had left Latvia and Lithuania when the Jews were banished after the assassination of the Czar. Her parents owned a grocery store in a small town. Even as a child she felt stifled by the small-mindedness, gossip, and disapproving eyes of her surroundings. She went to Emerson College on a scholarship to study broadcasting and theater and then returned to Richmond to employment as a radio show host. It was a man's world, and sexism limited her advancement. For instance, as a woman, Betty was not allowed to have any input in her own show.

Feeling suffocated, she left for New York City. She literally grabbed the midnight train on the spur of the moment with no clue as to what her future would bring. At first she supported herself as a barista and landed a few small roles in the theater. Before she could fulfill her dream to become a successful actress, she got married to an actor and had two children. She was a devoted mother but still worked to support the family and eventually became manager of the well-known Gaslight Café in Greenwich Village.

However, New York City was not the environment she wanted her children to grow up in. Eventually Betty relocated to Woodstock, New York, and found a community of artistic friends. There her children thrived. Betty felt rejuvenated surrounded by nature and began to feel truly at home. The community gave her a sense of belonging. She had found her tribe.

For well over 20 years, Betty has been involved with Playback Theater, a form of therapy that brings people's lives on stage to instill self-awareness. She works as a psychotherapist and simultaneously has found a variety of artistic expressions such as sculpting and multimedia art.

In Betty's own words: "I love growing old and continuing to learn."

Currently, Betty is working on her own book about the joys and complexities of aging.

Thomas Moore, psychotherapist and spiritual philosopher, defines a true community as "a gathering of individuals who can be open and free with each other without fear. In short, they can be themselves." Moore agrees with the English pediatrician and psychoanalyst D.W. Winnicott, who posited that the ability to play indicates psychological well-being, a sense of being real, and that "compliance is community's enemy." What did Winnicott mean by this? People, he says, sacrifice their authenticity for fear of not belonging or of not being accepted by a given community, whether it's a family, a high school clique, a fraternal organization, a company, or whatever the group may be. Winnicott felt that "compliance carries with it a sense of futility for the individual and is associated with the idea that nothing matters, and that life is not worth living."[9]

Pathfinder Daniel Klein wrote *Travels with Epicurus*, his meditation on aging, while spending a year on Hydra in the Greek islands. He was accepted into the local clan, the men hanging out at the tavern all day, philosophizing, drinking, and admiring the attractive young women who passed by. "I never had a strong relationship with my own father, who I observed, when not working, had no real friends or community," Klein confesses. His daily gathering of friends and comrades in Greece, he noticed, kept his juices moving. At home in Great Barrington, Massachusetts, Dan continues to lunch with friends. The camaraderie fans his creative fires while giving him a strong sense of community.

When we are children, we want desperately to belong, especially within our home, then our school, and so on. True community, like true belonging, begins with an individual's desire but is lived out through

---

[9] D. W. Winnicott, *Playing and Reality* (New York: Routledge, 1971), p. 65

connection with others. When older people have
healed, or at least accepted old childhood wounds, and
have held themselves accountable for wrongs they may
have committed, they can step beyond themselves and
approach others with compassion. This is easier said
than done within families, where mutual resonance
may be lacking. By contrast, in a chosen community of
like-minded souls, individuals thrive because they feel
free to express their true selves, basking in the warm
embrace of the group's acceptance.

Choosing Connection over Tradition

Historically, we are born into a family, and likely a
cultural community, whose values and morals we must
abide by in order to ensure our protection and social
support. Since we are social animals who need others
who will have our backs, we all too often accept mores
such as, "blood is thicker than water," even though
we may have little or no resonance with our blood
relations or the tribe of which they are a part.

Tribes originated on Earth in ancient times,
providing protection from the wild world. In
exchange for a sense of belonging, individuals often
declared loyalty and conceded to the group's rules and
guidelines. The roles of the group were clearly defined.
The elders commanded respect and deference. Because

the children were expected to carry on the work of the older generation, marriages were arranged to best serve the group. In turn, as they matured, the children took on more responsibility. Honoring aging was integral to the survival of the tribe. In every culture, when people reached 70, my age at this writing, they were considered old. The elders became role models for the younger generations. Through their day-to-day behavior, they demonstrated *how* to age.

I grew up in a traditional Jewish family where indeed the "blood bond" was the only option. Having fled Greece before the war or survived the concentration camps, their bond was written in stone. The sheer reality of the Holocaust left a visceral imprint on every family in our close-knit community. All the houses on our block in Brooklyn were from the same vacated village in Greece. This created a sense of security and belonging, where each family, each person, had the other's back.

Our community continued time-honored rituals, including celebration and prayers on all the holidays. But for me, and many in my generation, the rituals, although beautiful, felt devoid of meaning or true spirituality.

A teaching story called "The Guru's Cat" comes to mind:

When the guru sat down to worship each evening the ashram cat would get in the way and distract the worshippers. So he ordered that the cat be tied during evening worship.

After the guru died, the cat continued to be tied during evening worship. And when the cat expired, another cat was brought to the ashram so that it could be duly tied during evening worship.

Centuries later the guru's scholarly disciples wrote learned treatises on the liturgical significance of tying up a cat while worship is performed.

—Anthony de Mello, from *The Song of the Bird*

By the 1960s, youth in many Western cultures sought more independence and freedom of expression beyond the insular confines of the families that had raised them. In America, in particular, the frustration of a large segment of middle-class young people with the time-honored conventions imposed upon them by their parents and grandparents exploded into a cultural movement that broke barriers in civil rights, awakened sexual freedom, and gave women a new voice. The rising tide of shifting mores could not be denied. The traditional no longer dictated the behaviors necessary for survival—quite the contrary.

As I became a young adult, striking out on my

own in the turbulent 1960s, like many of my peers, I began to step away and create my own life. I was acutely aware that my friends had become my new tribe, that I could choose a "family" more in keeping with my nature. The free-spirited ethos of the time fueled our confidence.

In modern days we are free to *choose* our social group, as individual and group psychotherapist Daniel I. Malamud clarified in 1974 with his theory of the great benefit of the "second-chance family." I was privileged to work with him as he was working on this thesis. He believed that "the future holds a place for second-chance families in which main ties will be based not on birth or marital choice, but rather on members' commitment to seek together new opportunities for nourishment and challenge that they may not have had enough of in their actual childhood families." [10]

The goal is not to choose one or the other, but, if possible, to embrace both biological and social tribes. We may learn to "play certain games," but only if we are not sabotaging who we authentically are. We can even play those games consciously, according to R. D. Laing, who posed this profound insight:

[10] Daniel I. Malamud, *Journal of Humanistic Psychology*, Volume 14, No. 2, Spring, 1974.

"They are playing a game.

I see that they are playing a game.

If I show them I see that they are playing a game, I break the rules and they punish me.

Therefore, I must play the game of not seeing I see the game!"

We need our tribe, biological and social, particularly in this time of pandemic.

In America in particular, grown children live in other states and create "families" or "tribes" where they live based on what's important to them. In urban and rural communities alike, we tend to bond with those around us. If we can choose a tribe that fosters positive outlooks and like-mindedness, even sharing spiritual practices to maintain connection with the tribe and something beyond the tribe, life expectancies can actually expand.

In a 2018 cover story on aging, TIME magazine reported that for some people, maintaining connection with even their immediate family can be very challenging, especially as people age and families disperse. However, the article also cited a 2017 study in the journal *Personal Relationships* that offered promise to those who struggle with difficult family relationships: "It can be friends, not family, who matter most. The study looked at 270,000 people in nearly 100 countries and found that while both family and friends are associated with happiness and better health, as people aged, the health link remained only for people with strong friendships." [11]

Two of our Pathfinders, Iris Alster, 97, and Dr. Irving Milberg, 100, attested to the importance of family in their long lives. Iris considers her elder community of "wonderful, supportive friends" a "family" as well. Before he died at 100, Dr. Milberg told me that his family had become his passion: his wife, kids, grandchildren, and great grandchildren. I believed him, but I also knew that he loved to learn and never gave up on helping others heal. When I last spoke with Irving, he talked of hanging up his shingle. Knowing that he would be 100 in a few months, I laughed and cautioned him, "Don't make any rash decisions. Why not wait until you're a centenarian?"

Thriving Social Networks Enjoy Long and Healthy Lives

"The community stagnates without the impulse of the individual. The impulse dies without the sympathy of the community."

—William James

---

[11] Kluger, Jeffrey and Sifferlin, Alexandra, *"How To Live Longer, Better"* TIME magazine, 2/15/18, p. 48

In her book *Cure: A Journey into the Science of Mind and Body*, science journalist Jo Marchant discusses how societies with social networks thrive and enjoy longer and healthier lives.

She cites a 2005 study by Luis Rosero-Bixby, a demographer at the University of Costa Rica in San José, who used electoral records to determine Costa Ricans' life expectancies. Though typically people in the world's richest countries live the longest, he found that even though Costa Rica's per capita income is only about 20% of that of the U.S., if its residents survive the country's relatively high rates of infections and accidents early in life, they live exceedingly long—especially the men. Costa Rican men often live to be well over 100.

My wife and I recently visited the Nicoya peninsula, a gorgeous, diverse stretch of rainforest and open land that meets the Pacific Ocean on Costa Rica's northwest border, just south of the Nicaraguan border. We noticed how happy the people were and how they respected and honored their elders' wisdom.

One of Rosero-Bixby's studies reveals that Nicoyans exhibit a strong emotional bond with family and community. The prevalence of these deep connections safeguard Nicoyans from chronic stress that would otherwise undermine their extraordinary longevity. They are certainly poor, but the love among them appears to keep them young.

When we are interdependent, we share, but we cannot share until we realize that we alone do not know all the answers. No one individual or system of thought has a corner on all the wisdom available in the world. Wisdom comes from experience; it is revealed only when we have prepared ourselves to receive it, when we have opened our hearts. Ancient Chinese medicine teaches that the feminine soul of healing guides us, confirming that our strength comes not from self-absorption but from acknowledging our need for each other.

Lao-tzu's book of wisdom, the *Tao Te Ching*, emphasizes this inherently feminine nature of the Tao:

> *There was something formless and perfect*
> *before the universe was born.*
> *It is serene. Empty.*
> *Solitary. Unchanging.*
> *Infinite. Eternally present.*
> *It is the mother of the universe.*
> *For lack of a better name,*
> *I call it the Tao.*
> *It flows through all things,*
> *inside and outside, and returns*
> *to the origin of all things.*

In the 1970s, an American woman named Grace Halsell lived for two years among the Vilcabamban people of the Andes Mountains in Ecuador, well known for its large population of individuals in their 100s and wrote a book about her experiences. On why she believed the Vilcabambans lived well and long, Halsell writes:

"Living among the *viejos* (long-lived), I never heard them quarrel or fight or dispute with each other. They had what I would consider a 'high' culture in this regard. They spoke beautifully, elegantly, with ample flourishes of tenderness. Their words themselves were often caresses." [12]

Halsell attributed the health and harmony of the Vilcabambato to the strength of their community, where all ages interrelated with one another.

Somewhat like extended families in America before the Industrial Revolution, the Vilcabambans relished all the benefits and comforts that come from reciprocally sharing one's life with loved ones.

"In 2010, U.S. researchers analyzed 148 studies following more than 308,000 people and concluded that lacking strong social bonds doubles the risk of death from all causes....In Western societies, at least,

---

[12] Grace Halsell, *Los Viejos: Secrets of Long Life from the Sacred Valley* (Rodale Books, 1976), p. 13.

social isolation is as harmful as drinking and smoking, and suggests that it is actually more dangerous than lack of exercise or obesity.

When we have social support, we live more healthily…People who have warm relationships, rich social lives, and who feel like they are embedded in a group 'don't get as sick, and they live longer,' says Charles Raison, a psychiatry professor and mind–body medicine researcher at the University of Wisconsin–Madison. 'It's probably the single most powerful behavioral finding in the world.'" [13]

In one of my favorite modern teaching stories, a simple man known as Jacob the Baker affirms the need to unite together in order to overcome our fear and confusion:

> *A neighbor of Jacob's needed to start on a journey, but it was the middle of the night.*
>
> *Afraid to begin, afraid not to begin…he came to Jacob.*
>
> *"There is no light on the path," he complained.*
>
> *"Take someone with you," counseled Jacob.*
>
> *"Jacob, what do you mean? If I do that, there will be two blind men."*
>
> *"You are wrong," said Jacob. "If two people discover each other's blindness, it is already growing light."*

---

[13] Jo Marchant, *Cure: A Journey into the Science of Mind Over Body* (Crown Publishers: New York, 2016) p. 179-181.

Loneliness and the Brain

In the midst of our current pandemic, we must face the reality of social isolation. This makes reaching out even more difficult. For in our isolation, we feel more helpless and hopeless. But, we must take the initiative and ask for help or help ourselves by helping others. This is the time to forgive old grudges and trust that connection is available to us even without contact and touch.

Note: Refer to the end of this chapter, under "Cultivating the Seeds," where lifesaving strategies appear for you to try.

For most of human history when individuals become separated from others, particularly from their "tribe," they become vulnerable to both attack by predators and to starvation. We all know how horrible it feels to be left out, ridiculed and ostracized. Study after study show that loneliness and isolation are more detrimental to health and longevity than the more obvious indicators like diet, exercise, education, or religious affiliation.

The efficacy of the brain's prefrontal cortex—which regulates self-awareness, rational thought, and social behavior—diminishes more swiftly than other parts of the brain. This can lead to dementia, particularly in those who are lonely and chronically stressed. This essential part of the brain regulates self-awareness, rationality, and social behavior.

Through her research, Michelle Carlson, PhD, a neuroscientist at the Johns Hopkins Bloomberg School of Public Health, hoped to slow that deterioration. Knowing that older people tend to isolate and become lonely as they age, particularly after retirement or losing a life partner, Dr. Carlson decided to experiment with exposing such folks to a vibrant social setting. She developed a project called Experience Corps, in which elderly adults spend 15 hours each week volunteering in beleaguered elementary schools, helping kids with their reading. Typically volunteers don't last at such programs, but this elder group stayed with it through the entire academic year. Both patient and wise, they were able to imagine what these troubled children may be living with at home, and they truly wanted them to succeed. They formed very close relationships with the children—a kind of magical connection that may be lacking with teachers or even parents. "We tell them we need them, their wisdom and experience," Carson noted. "They do it not for themselves but because the kids are waiting for them.…They really can sometimes connect with the child on a different level."[14]

---

[14] Ibid. p. 189.

The Experience Corps program markedly improved both the children's academic achievement and also the volunteers' health. "It was like watering them," added Carlson. A pilot trial published in 2009 suggested that over the school year the volunteers' overall activity increased and their legs got considerably stronger, both of which usually decline with age. Their performance on cognitive tests also improved, and the activity in their prefrontal cortex increased. [15]

These studies validate the theory that the social network encourages a positive relationship with aging and substantiates the importance of rightly choosing our tribe.

Cultivating the Seeds of the Second Grace: Finding Your Tribe

To nourish the seeds of the second grace, the importance of relationships for conscious aging and finding one's tribe, these guidelines may help shift any residual belief that old people spend their days alone, lonely, sad, and waiting to die.

1. **Engage in conversation**, make contact with people when you're out doing your errands—the clerk, the bus driver, whoever you find around you. Look for opportunities to be kind.

---

[15] Ibid. p. 190.

2. **Give extra energy to deepening sincere friendships.** Consider who is a true friend and who is not. Studies show that just one good friend can improve health and promote longevity. Don't feed relationships that tend to drain you, or in which you feel regularly criticized—such "friendships" can be toxic.

3. **Nurture biological family relationships,** if possible. These offer many benefits, including shared history, shared memories, and hopefully love.

4. **View learning as a lifelong endeavor.** Enroll in courses or workshops that interest you. This also provides opportunities to expand your social network. For continuing education, explore local college, public library and community center programs and events, as well as senior centers.

5. **Don't sell yourself short.** Find groups who appreciate and accept you, as you are, who don't demand that you conform to their standards. We can more readily take constructive criticism from those who accept us, rather than those who judge us. Plus, creating new friendships comes naturally when you're involved in a shared endeavor with accepting people.

6. **Get involved and give back.** Explore possibilities with which you may resonate. Scan

your local paper as well as the bulletin board at your local public library or community college. Search online. If you don't find an opportunity that speaks to you, consider creating one.

7. **Volunteer.** Day care centers, primary schools, and pediatric wards in hospitals, for example, are always in need of loving caregivers. The reciprocity of giving loving attention offers often-unexpected rewards.

8. **When you feel lonely, reach out** and call a friend.

Online Resources for Finding Your Tribe

Gray Is Green is an online gathering of older adult Americans aspiring to create a green legacy for the future. http://grayisgreen.org

If you want to live forever, these are the Best Counties To Live In: https://www.realtor.com/news/trends/best-counties-want-live-forever?cid=prt_patch_editorial_web_move

How about "Nightclub action" for seniors? https://www.vice.com/en_uk/article/j5az48/this-nightclub-for-the-elderly-is-fighting-loneliness-with-tea-party-raves

Want to Meet Up?: http://www.meetup.com

Why Communes May Be the New Retirement Home: https://huffingtonpost/entry/communes-may-be-the-new-retirement-home_us_55e47693e4b0b7a9633994476

University-based retirement communities: https://www.aplaceformom.com/blog/9-3-14-seniors-head-back-to-school/

Quirky Retirement Communities: https://www.marketwatch.com/story/8-quirky-retirement-communities-2013-01-22?page=1

How To Find Friends and Fight Loneliness:

https://sixtyandme.com/how-to-find-friends-and-fight-loneliness-after-60/

Volunteer Abroad For Seniors and Retirees:

https://www.volunteerforever.com/article_post/volunteer-abroad-opportunities-for-seniors-and-retirees

https://www.travelandleisure.com/syndication/volunteer-jobs-retirement-best-perks

Elders taking action: https://eldersaction.org

Wisdom and Spirit in Action:

https://www.sage-ing.org

THIRD GRACE

Practicing Mindfulness

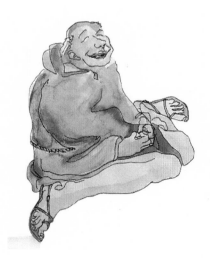

To see a World in a Grain of Sand
And a Heaven in a Wild Flower,
Hold Infinity in the palm of your hand
And Eternity in an hour.
—William Blake, from "Auguries of Innocence"

"Water....flows on and on, and merely fills up all the
places through which it flows; it does not shrink from any
dangerous spot nor from any plunge, and nothing can make
it lose its own essential nature. It remains true to itself
under all conditions."
—*The I Ching, Book of Changes*

"The older one gets the more one feels that the present
must be enjoyed, it is a precious gift, comparable to a state
of grace."
—Scientist Marie Curie

"Aging doesn't bother me. You breathe in and out. I have
always felt as if I lived on a lily pond and life gives me
its abundance."
—Pathfinder Iris Alster

"I have become totally comfortable living in the unknown."
—Pathfinder Sarnie Ogus

"How can you think and hit at the same time!"
—Yogi Berra

IRIS ALSTER
——— AGE 97 ———

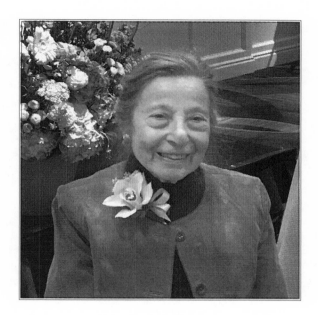

Iris Alster lives a mindful life. She would not need to name it so, and would be surprised to open this chapter on mindfulness and find her own story. She hasn't studied mindfulness, yet her innate awareness continues to nurture her long life.

Iris lived through many hard times. Born and raised in Brooklyn in a family that had escaped oppression in Europe, young Iris experienced the Great Depression, her father's bankruptcy, and her family's existential struggles. She could not pursue her dream of going to college, but instead went to a secretarial school, one of the few options available to Jewish women at that time. The U.S. Navy hired her as a secretary, which led Iris to the opportunity to train as a nurse.

She worked for many years at Bellevue Hospital in New York City and became involved in caring for the homeless. Invited by one of the medical professors to become a private nurse in his practice, Iris jumped at the chance. She remained a loyal member of the doctor's staff for 40 years, following him to North Carolina, where he had become dean of a medical school.

Iris married but never had children, and her husband died young. When I interviewed her, she remarked, "My life has been like floating on a lily pad."

There is no caution in her optimism, no resentment, no regret, no bitterness, or stinginess. She insists that good things continue to manifest in her life, and she feels deeply grateful, knowing no greater joy than giving back.

Iris became my patient about ten years ago at age 86. Her primary motivation for acupuncture treatment was, in her words, "to stay connected to my vitality." She takes no medication and has no complaints.

Iris's greatest gifts are her infectious joy, her adventurous spirit, her playfulness, and her naturally deep spirituality, which she never speaks about but clearly lives.

Iris travelled to Tibet in her seventies, which left her with "an inexplicable something, a connection to something deeper." She travelled to Burma at the age of 91 and has no plans of stopping her adventures.

She has always led and still leads a life of service, which she considers her true source of vitality and joy. Iris now lives in an elder community that encourages independent living. She considers this community her tribe. She loves the intellectual stimulation, daily yoga, and classes, but mostly she enjoys her companions and her sense of community. To this day Iris is as effervescent as ever.

ANDREW FERBER M.D.
——— AGE 86 ———

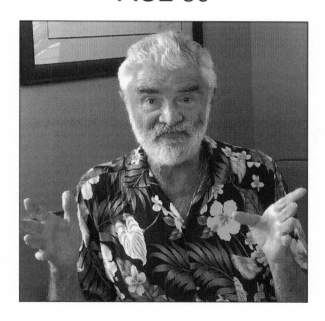

*Both of **Andrew Ferber**'s parents were the children of immigrants. Both his father and his paternal grandfather*

were physicians. His mother helped run a small grocery. For as long as Andrew can remember, his parents never let him forget about the harshness and prejudice that exist in the world. "You're Jewish, they'll give you nothing, you must stand strong!" they admonished their son. Naturally, young Andrew became sensitized to issues of social injustice. By the time he reached adulthood, he was drawn to a career path devoted to helping combat these problems.

Andrew went to medical school, specializing in Psychiatry. He manifested his passion for life by learning how to help others and became the youngest professor of Psychiatry at the Albert Einstein College of Medicine, an institution committed to social equality and healthcare devoted to all that upholds the qualities of its namesake. A perfect place for Andrew to thrive. He authored books and numerous articles by the time he reached his thirties. He married a fellow physician and became a father, doing everything he was supposed to do to create an "ideal" life. Still, Andrew felt there was something missing.

Working in medicine made Andrew acutely aware of mortality, his own and everyone else's. Western medicine had its limitations, he believed, and his passion for meditation grew, adding a lifelong spiritual component to his psychiatric practice.

Andrew's spiritual studies took him to India where he was given the name Swami Bodhicitta. He is currently at work on a book and creating teaching seminars on the Tibetan Bardo, the study of the gap between death and rebirth, the

*Tibetan art of living and dying. At 86, the medical director
of Chrysalis Health, he remains in private practice.*

*For over 50 years Andrew has studied and taught
meditation. He returns to India each year to revitalize his
spiritual practice. Bodhicitta embodies the Seven Graces
of Ageless Aging. He eats only organic, vegetarian food,
exercises and practices yoga daily, taps into his passion, and
has no intention of ever retiring!*

The mind can heal, and the mind can slay.
Whether serving us or not, our intentions, our fears, our
preoccupations, our obstacles, and our obsessions can
run away with us, unless we are present to our choices,
our actions, and our experiences. The mind creates
illusions of past and future whereas simply being in
the present involves the here and now. For the sake of
clarity, let's define "mindfulness" as being receptive to
the present moment, in mind and body, noticing what
passes before us, witnessing our life, without judgment.

In the First Grace, Rewriting the Script, we
considered the power of the mind and how our beliefs
and even our thoughts can impact our health and the
aging process. We learned that when we focus our
intentional mind like a laser, we can affect reality. The
Third Grace, Practicing Mindfulness, is not about
directing the mind, but about learning to be present,

allowing, in essence, the absence of thought, or the ability to observe thought in a detached way.

This old story from the Aegean islanders told in Daniel Klein's *Travels with Epicurus* illustrates how we defer to our programmed beliefs rather than noticing, being mindful in our lives:

An affluent Greek American man, visiting the islands, is out for a walk. He comes upon an old Greek man sitting on a rock, sipping ouzo, wistfully staring into the sea as the sun sets. The American notices the untended olive trees growing on the hillside behind the man, olives dropping to the ground. He approaches the old Greek man and asks who owns the olive trees.

"I do," the Greek man replies.

"Don't you harvest your olives?" the American asks.

"I just pick one or two when I want to."

"But don't you realize that if you cared for the trees, pruned them, and picked them when they're ready, you could sell them? Everyone loves virgin olive oil; they pay a good price for a bottle in America."

"What would I do with the money?"

"You could build a big house and hire servants to do your work."

"And then what would I do?"

"You could do anything you wanted to do."

"You mean, like sit outside, sipping ouzo while the sun sets?"

The Third Grace focuses on studies, techniques, and guidelines to help create and sustain a mindful life. In fact, individuals who practice mindfulness live a fuller, richer, and longer life. They often experience life as a spiritual or soul journey. People who feel spiritually connected are not necessarily religious, but feel connected to the universe, the cosmic current, and all of its lessons. Such people experience a spacious contentment, which can increase their lifespan.

To begin a meditative practice, I often encourage my clients to develop an inner witness, a "watcher on the hill," who is always available to them. This watching, however, can occur on two planes of consciousness: 1) the witness who observes oneself without judgment and 2) the ego, who watches and judges. The witness practices self-awareness while self-consciousness drives the ego. Simply try to watch yourself, your reactions, your fear, and happiness from a position of detachment. Say to yourself, "this too will pass."

My friend and mindfulness trainer, Douglas Scherer, Ed.D., teaches that in order to be truly mindful we must change our relationship to "now," noticing and allowing, without striving for perfection. He suggests that we can even approach the aches and pains of aging with curiosity, with a beginner's mind. This creates spaciousness, even ease, within us, allowing the pain to dissolve naturally.

Spiritual Eldering

"If your mind is empty, it is always ready for anything; it is open to everything. In the beginner's mind there are many possibilities, but in the expert's, there are few."
—**Shunryu Suzuki**

Rabbi Schachter-Shalomi coined the concept of spiritual eldering, meaning to focus in later life on spiritual development, interpersonal relationships, communication, and service and to model these practices for others. He believed that spiritual eldering goes hand in hand with consciousness, embracing the potential of the mind and the ability to be mindful.

We use only a small percentage of our brain's capacity. When we live a long life, our brain has the potential to further evolve, particularly when we practice mindfulness and cultivate our intuition. Enhancing our intuitive capacities, that is, our nonlinear perceptions, opens us more readily to the invisible or sacred realms, fostering mystical experiences, artistic inspiration, and scientific discovery. Rabbi Schachter-Shalomi suggests that creativity once belonging only to great artists, scientists, philosophers, and mystics, can become a learned skill available to many people.

"Conventional religion often fulfills people's need for social belonging. How different this is from spiritual eldering, which deals with developing contemplative skills, harvesting one's life, leaving a legacy for the future, and preparing for death. It's the difference between seeking safety and comfort, on the one hand, and reducing the ego and opening to the Spirit, on the other. The religious elder says, 'I want to be saved. I want to remain safe and secure in my religious identity. I don't want to feel the anxiety of facing the unknown.' The spiritual elder says, 'I want to work on myself, even if that means facing past and present anxieties. I want to be generous, pure, and clean in facing the Spirit. I want to live the truth as I see it.'" [16]

In *Ordinarily Sacred*, author Lynda Sexson clarifies the true meaning of religion: "(It) is not a discrete category within human experience; it is rather a quality that pervades all experience."

We know this true meaning in our bones when we traverse the boundaries of conventional thought and feelings and enter the domain of deep mystery within and beyond everything we experience.

Transcending Stereotypes

> *"Perfection is spelled PARALYSIS."*
>
> **—Sir Winston Churchill**

Control is a relative thing. We cannot change what happens to us, but we can control our responses and reactions to whatever life delivers. Our beliefs either

---

[16] Zalman Schachter-Shalomi and Ronald S. Miller, *From Age-ing to Sage-ing: A Revolutionary Approach to Growing Older* (New York: Grand Central Publishing, 2014), p. 40.

foster self, allowing us to be centered, or obliviate our connection to our root, putting us at the mercy of outside influences.

When older adults embrace negative stereotypes of expected decline, they not only create self-fulfilling prophecies, but also activate negative neural pathways in the brain, making it more and more likely that they will repeat the automatic, unconscious behavior. In turn, one person's negative expectations about aging can also influence another's, such as in long-term marriages, which can create an inter-relational fulfilling prophecy. Such a dynamic also encourages and can perpetuate one partner's dependency on the other or co-dependency, both of which can create a sense of losing control, which can precipitate breakdowns in physical and emotional health. Mindfulness supports our ability to be present in the moment, which grounds us in our experience, providing more control of external stimuli.

Research reveals that believing one is in control is more important than actually being in control. Handicapped or elderly people, who struggle with physical limitations, may learn to be helpless, essentially giving up control of their care to others, particularly deferring to physicians, nurses, and long-term caregivers. Belief in one's capacities can, in fact, improve one's self-confidence and therefore one's physical, mental, and emotional health.

Health care institutions often foster the very negative stereotypes that keep the elderly down by perpetuating a climate of dependency. We may wonder who is controlling whom. Such behavior not only diminishes an elder's integrity and sense of self, it can literally cause misdiagnosis and reduce treatment options that can seriously impact health outcomes.

The cultural perpetuation of such negative stereotypes increases the perception that with age, one's identity, who one is and has been, will dissipate with shifts in ability, possibilities, or outlook for the future. Elinor Langer asks, for example, is a painter no longer a painter if he or she cannot hold a brush?

By the age of 50, Pierre Auguste Renoir, the French Impressionist painter, began to suffer from crippling rheumatoid arthritis, but he kept painting, finding ways to cope. Even when he could not hold a brush, he would bind his hand in a soft cloth and have the brush placed within it. His strokes became broader with more sweep but no less vivid in color and emotion. When Henri Matisse met with Renoir in his older years, he commented, "As his body dwindled, the soul in him seemed to grow stronger continually and express itself with more radiant ease."

Apparently Renoir understood that the aging process means change, bringing with it limitations and loss, but he seemed to know that the self is not defined by our activities but rather by the nature of our soul and its eternal longing. Life is a continuum. When older individuals (all of us!) are able to mindfully expand their understanding of what defines them, embracing the continuity of life, they realize that they are who they have always been.

My client and friend, Pathfinder Gillian Jagger, the artist and sculptor, continued making art well into older age, as she had done successfully since the 1960s. Complications from a fall brought on her death in November 2019.

Gillian told me that what she most appreciated about making art was that with each piece of sculpture she created, she felt she was expressing herself for the first time. The creative process kept her innocent and excited. She said it was a great relief to no longer be self-conscious. "My work need not say something intelligent. It just is," she declared. She believed that authentic art uses the artist as a medium through whom the art comes alive.

Since 1985, Jagger brought "found life" into the studio. The objects she chose point to the essential, significant forms that repeat through time in nature—meandering, spiraling, branching, and cracking. In her most recent work, she asked, "How do I follow nature rather than trying to make it do something? I know I've captured the essence of what I'm intending when I fully experience it myself." Her mindfulness, she believed, allowed the work to come through her.

I have found it endlessly valuable to mindfully observe those elders in my life who continue to live full lives. Many of them are the Pathfinders cited throughout this book. When we pay attention to others' behavior, we not only learn from them, they receive positive reinforcement from us.

Embracing Impermanence

In our American culture that often celebrates the young and casts off its old, the fact of impermanence, of certain death, often challenges the old to hold onto their vanished youth. Think of the old woman whose hands reveal her age but her Botoxed face has no wrinkles. It's unnatural at least, and some would say desacralizes the body, the natural growing younger towards death. Some cultures celebrate wrinkles on an old face as the signs of richly earned experience, the roadmap of a life well lived. We will all leave our bodies one day. What if we could embrace our waning physique and see the beauty behind the façade?

There is a great peace inherent in simply being, a state in which what we do is less important than simply being who we are.

This reminds me of an old favorite joke:

Two men bump into each other on the street and realize that their sons used to be good friends.

"So how's your boy Joey?" one asks.

"He can't seem to hold on to a job, can't find a good relationship! I hope he finds his way. How is Steven doing?"

The other father looks up and explains, "He's doing yoga, is into health food, and has discovered meditation! At least he's DOING something!"

In *This is Getting Old: Zen Thoughts on Aging with Humor & Dignity*, Susan Moon shares the story of a dharma sister, someone who, after 35 years of diligent Zen practice and service, developed Alzheimer's and began to struggle in her relations with family and friends. When she stayed close to the Zen center, however, and her practice, she remained totally present, meditative, and could simply be. Her beingness took her out of her mind and into the present moment.

A friend told me a similar story about visiting a beloved mentor who had begun to show serious signs of dementia. She seemed herself though she did not recognize the former students who had come to visit her. When they engaged her, however, in memories of their study together, she brightened and tapped into the self that her students had known. Her eyes glistened with aliveness and her ability to be fully present shone through. She did not have to think about it; she *was* it!

Derived from a Buddhist teaching, "'wabi-sabi' is a Japanese expression for the beauty of impermanence, the imperfection of things that are worn or frayed or chipped through use. Objects that are simple and rustic, like an earthenware tea-bowl, and objects that show their age and use, like a wooden bannister worn smooth by many hands are beautiful." [17]

There's also the story of the Zen potter who had crafted the perfect bowl but finding no imperfections became very upset, unable to consider his work acceptable. He chose instead to break the perfect bowl and glue it back together to give it the true beauty that he had envisioned through its imperfect being.

I'm remembering an evening at the Rubin Museum in New York that also illustrates inevitable impermanence. I watched, mesmerized, as a group of Tibetan monks completed a gorgeous floor painting with colored sands that they had created over many weeks. They prayed over it, honoring its grand beauty, and then ceremoniously scattered the sand, laughing all the while, as a metaphoric celebration of impermanence.

This story illustrates that in its continual transformation from one state to another, the world is exactly as it should be:

> *Many years ago a woman called Sono lived in a little town in Japan. Her devout heart and compassionate spirit had won her the respect and admiration of many followers, and fellow Buddhists often travelled long distances to seek her advice. One day a weary*

[17] Susan Moon, *This is Getting Old: Zen Thoughts on Aging with Humor & Dignity* (Shambala Publications: Boston, 2010) p. xii

traveler approached Sono to ask what he could do to put his mind at peace and his heart at rest.

Sono's advice was simple and straightforward: "In the morning and in the evening, whenever anything occurs to you, say, "Thanks for everything. I have no complaint whatsoever!"

For an entire year the man faithfully followed her advice, repeating from morning until evening, "Thanks for everything. I have no complaint whatsoever!" But still his mind was not at peace nor was his heart at rest. Thoroughly discouraged, he again made the long journey to see Sono. "I've done everything you suggested," he said, "but my mind is not at peace and my heart is not at rest. Tell me— what should I do now?"

As Sono replied, "Thanks for everything. I have no complaint whatsoever!"

Hearing these words the traveler was enlightened and returned home, his mind at peace and his heart at rest.

Mindfulness and Stress

"Flow with whatever may happen and let your mind be free. Stay centered by accepting whatever you are doing. This is the ultimate."

—Chuang Tzu

For half a century, physiologists have known that animals under stress age very quickly. In human beings too, the accumulated results of stress look very much like growing old. Older people, too, recover much less quickly from stressful situations, often depleted by exhaustion. Deepak Chopra notes that "one year of old age produces as much deterioration in the stress response as two years of middle age…eventually, the instinct to come back into balance breaks down completely, and even mild stresses—a bout of flu, a minor fall, losing a small amount of money—become extremely difficult to cope with." [18] This situation can create a perpetual feeling of "helplessness/hopelessness," both prevalent in the elderly and often arising out of the expectation of a bad outcome, most notably due to memories. "There would be no stress without the memory of stress, for our memories dictate what frightens us or makes us angry. The curse of memory is that it ages us from the inside; our inner world is getting older, shutting us out from reality, which is never old." [19]

To restore and rejuvenate our bodies, as we grow older, we must inhibit the creation of hormones that can age us before our time. When we over-control our lives, bracing at the slightest hint of chaos or disappointment, we unnecessarily manufacture and release hormones such as cortisol and adrenaline that make matters worse. We can choose to go lightly, accepting everyday annoyances as part of life, allowing for more spontaneity

[18] Deepak Chopra, M.D. *Ageless Body, Timeless Mind: The Quantum Alternative to Growing Old* (Three Rivers Press: New York) p. 151
[19] Ibid. p. 157

and surprise. Rather than fretting over the latest "breaking news" and overscheduling our time with things that don't bring us joy, we can put joy on our calendars in the form of exercise, meditation, journaling, listening to music, gardening, or taking a walk in nature. In short, by consciously letting go of trying to control the external world, we regain an internal control by accepting what is.

To activate this wisdom in one form or another asks us to be mindful, to cultivate an inner witness that perceives our best remedy in the moment and to employ it. The mind is very powerful, able to manufacture chemicals every second with each thought we make. The release of the stress hormone, cortisol, for example, secreted by the adrenal glands can negatively impact health and promote aging. On the other hand, mindfulness can reduce, temper, and even eliminate such negative effects of stress. What better time to learn these skills, both young and old, considering the constant stressors that plague every aspect of our lives!

There are many current studies that substantiate the theory that stress in older people can be reduced through mindfulness—living in the present, right here, right now. This simple practice can be applied instantly, moment to moment, hour to hour, day to day. Research attests to the positive effects of mindfulness in the alleviation of excess worry. Worry projects past hurt into the future. When we become present to the moment, worry dissipates.

Sometimes the mindful act of reframing worry by casting it in a positive light can relieve our stress. Consider this story:

An old man was bitter and challenged Jacob with a complaint.

"All my life I have searched for meaning," he said.

"The meaning is in the search," said Jacob, waving off the man's distress.

"Then I will never find the meaning?"

"No," said Jacob. "You will never stop looking."

Jacob held his voice for a moment, unsure if he had been too harsh.

"My friend," Jacob began again, "know that you are a man with a lantern who goes in search of a light."

This story speaks to our Pathfinder David Lewine's experience.

David Lewine, 86, whose story I share in the chapter on the Fifth Grace: Pursuing Your Passion, is an excellent example of "reframing," that is, finding his true calling, through art and mindfulness. After several disastrous turns in his life in order to find stability, often to no avail, he finally set out on a new path that connected his strengths and passions with service for the greater good. At a critical point in his life he beat a bout of depression by finding his connection to music and learning to play the guitar. Art led him to meditation and yoga. His passions grew and deepened, and for the last 50 years, David has combined his love of meditation and music with teaching. Today he lives in the service of Karma Yoga, also known as the art of compassion.

Meditation Practice as an Antidote to Stress

Meditation directly addresses the root of the stress response. It releases memories of stress and lowers levels of cortisol and adrenaline in the body. Studies have shown that Transcendental Meditation (TM), Primordial Sound Meditation, and other meditative practices, can relieve the mind of thoughts and open to the silence below the thought, ultimately reaching "pure awareness," which exists between thoughts.

In 1978, R. Keith Wallace, a UCLA physiologist, began to research how meditation affects aging. He found that blood pressure, vision, and hearing—markers of aging—improved with long-term meditation practice and actually reversed the biological age.

Of course, meditation too can support a spiritual practice that seeks to unify one's body, mind, and spirit in balanced wholeness.

It is worth noting that choosing a meditation practice is not a "one size fits all" choice. In order to naturally discipline oneself to a practice, it is best to truly resonate with the chosen type of meditation. For one individual, silent sitting may resonate, for another walking quietly in nature works. In my book

Chinese Medicine for Maximum Immunity, I explore, for
example, the most appropriate forms of meditation for
the five Chinese elemental types: Wood, Fire, Earth,
Metal, and Water. I associate each with an archetype to
initially help individuals identify the type with which
they most resonate. Wood expresses the energy of the
Commander; Fire, the Lover; Earth, the Peacemaker;
Metal, the Artist, and Water, the Philosopher. Wood
types, who tend to have difficulty sitting still, do best
practicing an active meditation, such as tai chi or quiet
creative work. Fire types, whose energy can run rampant,
need the calming meditation of deep breathing. Earth
types, who can be sluggish, may benefit from meditative
free movement to an exhilarating piece of music.
Metal types, who tend to seek higher truth or moral
order, respond well to Zen meditation that involves the
willingness to let go and experience the wonder of being.
Simple, traditional meditation that quiets the mind by
focusing on the ingoing and outgoing breath, appeals
to Water types, who often long for silence, solitude, and
spiritual growth.

Mindfulness and Chronic Pain

Like anxiety and fear, we want as quickly as
possible to eliminate chronic pain. Paying non-
judgmental attention to chronic pain, without worry,
only observation, can create spaciousness in one's body
that actually eases pain.

Dr. Jon Kabat-Zinn found this to be true when he had his patients resist their temptation to eradicate their pain in favor of simply observing it. While anxiety and fear consist of many triggers, such as physical sensations, memories, imagined future outcomes, and repetitive internal narratives, chronic pain is usually related to a specific condition. Therefore when we focus on observing the language of the pain rather than on the recurring anxiety or fear that accompanies it, we realize that it is less complicated and probably more manageable. At the very least, when we can quiet our anxiety and fear, we allow our body to relax and listen more directly to the wisdom of the body and the mind.

This timeless Sufi teaching story illustrates this important point:

Mulla Nasreddin decided to create a flower garden. He prepared the soil and planted the seeds of many beautiful flowers. When the seeds sprouted and grew, along with his chosen flowers came an abundance of dandelions. He sought advice from many gardeners far and wide and tried every method known to get rid of dandelions, but to no avail. Finally he walked all the way to the Capitol to speak to the royal gardener at the Sheik's palace. The wise old man had counseled many gardeners before and suggested a variety of remedies to expel the dandelions, but Mulla had tried them all. They sat together in silence for some time until the royal gardener looked at Nasreddin and said, "Well then, I suggest you learn to love them!"

Leaning into Discomfort

Older individuals more often than not experience some form of chronic pain. The pharmaceutical industry and Western medicine's response to pain is to stop it, usually with medication that fogs the mind, numbs the nervous system, and can, in fact, become addictive.

What if rather than succumbing to yet another suggested prescription, we leaned into the pain, to experience it consciously, and even perhaps to kvetch about it? John Leland began writing *Happiness Is a Choice You Make* wondering how older people get through their days, particularly as they suffer with painful bodies and painful memories. He learned how the six elderly individuals he got to know for his book coped. Leland found through their stories that for the most part they embraced their suffering—not without complaint, demand, humor, or holding grudges— ultimately offering the author a transformational education in how to be resilient and to seek and find joy in daily life. He learned from these intrepid elders that even when inching toward 90 or even 100, we can have a remarkable impact on our life, particularly if "happiness is the choice we make."

Furthermore, when we embrace our suffering— the grave loss of a beloved, a crippled body, a forgetful mind—we choose to release our fear, our anxiety, our sorrow, which creates an inner spaciousness that broadens our perspective, often generating hope and even gratitude.

At 93, Pathfinder Sarnie Ogus, my early Alexander trainer introduced previously, attributes her long life to her mindful attitude and practice of Buddhism. She lives in a state of gratefulness. Each morning when she rises, she looks up and marvels, "Oh, I am so very grateful to be alive." "Realizing that I could take responsibility for my own suffering," she told me, "changed my life, changed my thinking about my place in the world."

A long-time client, Pathfinder Iris Alster, 97, who was introduced at the beginning of this chapter, was a former nurse. She attributes her long life to remaining open to everything. She believes that every moment is a celebration, a gift. She lives a mindful life by noticing and appreciating every detail.

"Tuning in" is essential to living mindfully, says Pathfinder Andrew Ferber (Bodhicitta,) a psychiatrist and spiritual teacher. He believes that wisdom resides in each of us. "We know when we're on or off the beam," he said in our interview. "I share similar advice with my clients about staying tuned in, present, mindful, to what feels right for them, at every level, and to honor that. Trusting that belief has certainly been my guide since an early age. From there we can take full responsibility for ourselves and our lives. We must practice self-inquiry. I say be evermore aware of yourself and trust what you find!"

Bodhichitta went on to share that he "believes that so much of illness is self-hatred. I've come to see that from the beginning, from perhaps the experiences in the womb, but definitely the initial experiences with the mother, the child develops a good self and a bad self. The bad self feels that, for example, 'I didn't get fed because I didn't deserve it' or 'I didn't get hugged because I'm bad.' This undeserving self gets bigger and bigger and remarkably people hold on to this idea well into adulthood because they believe that the bad self is who they are. If they let go of this idea, they don't exist. They'd rather hold on to the bad self than to be nobody. To help people love themselves, I encourage them to let go of the unloved self gradually. I tell them that loving yourself is natural. If it's difficult, there is a thought in the way. Wherever such thoughts occur, I encourage my clients to have fun, let go. I ask them to consider changing their erroneous thoughts, for example, "Who would you be if you loved yourself?"

In *Travels with Epicurus*, author and philosopher Daniel Klein reminds us that one of the gifts of aging is that things slow down; we can't move as fast. When you feel, for example, that you're falling behind, why not reframe that thought? Notice instead the life you are living, the simple pleasures of your existence. All of our senses, for instance, come to life when we become aware of them, when we notice, when we are mindful. We might say, we become aware of our awareness.

Michael Pollan illustrates this thought further in his latest book, *How To Change Your Mind: The New Science of Psychedelics*, where he cites research using psychedelic therapy, particularly psilocybin derived from magic mushrooms, to shift depression and thwart addictions to alcohol, cigarettes, and even cocaine. Psilocybin lifts the mind out of self-referential attachment to the ego and offers individuals a transcendent experience that they do not soon forget. This ultimate awareness awakens the mind like a mystical experience, leading to a better understanding of how the mind works while also offering a tool for changing it.

Cultivating the Seeds of the Third Grace: Practicing Mindfulness

1. **Develop your witness:** When we begin to witness our behavior, our actions, and that which happens around us, free from judgment, simply noticing, our life slows down. At first we become easily distracted but with practice, we notice the witness, now and again. As Ram Dass reminds us in *Polishing the Mirror*: "The witness is always here and now. It resides in each instant of living."

2. **Observe your breath:** When we allow our busy minds to rest, we ease into inhabiting our bodies, where true presence resides. We call

on our mind's attention to remind us of the great value of presence. We call in the witness and give ourselves time to simply be. The most common gateway to a meditative state uses the breath as guide, to rest upon, inhaling and exhaling with one's natural rhythm. If sitting meditation is not your cup of tea, you may prefer a walking meditation, listening to the surrounding sounds, again, allowing your mind to rest and your senses to quicken. These days wonderful podcasts offer a variety of meditations. Guided ones can be a gentle morning practice to get you started. The key is your choice to commit to the practice.

3. **Use visualizations:** For example: Find a comfortable chair or lie down. Allow your body to relax while maintaining your alertness. Release the tension in each joint and invite any tight or uncomfortable area in your body to release. Inhale light and exhale your tension. Lengthen your exhale. Allow the breath to be full and deep, emphasizing the exhale to expel all the air. Breathe in naturally through the nose, a full deep breath into your lungs. As you practice, imagine the light dissolving all of the oxidizing free radicals in your body, even if you don't know what they are.

4. **Practice sensory awareness:** As Charlotte Selver, the founder of the study of Sensory

Awareness and its foundation, so aptly put it, "There is something very sacred about our nature and the nature of things—the nature of coming together, being together, getting in contact with each other and having a sensitive connection to what we are doing." Sensory awareness is just what she says, bringing our awareness to our senses, particularly as mindfulness of the body. We can use our vision, our hearing, our smell, taste, and touch to connect to the world around us, *strictly* through our senses. As the saying goes, "Stop and smell the roses," but also touch them, enjoy their beauty as well as their imperfections, without judgment.

5. **Join a yoga class, a tai chi class, or a meditation or prayer group.** Such groups not only help to develop meditation skills, but also can serve as the Second Grace: Finding Your Tribe, by connecting you with a spiritually minded community.

6. **Go slowly and be present**, as the Buddhists say. When eating, eat; when drinking, drink; when playing, play. Lose yourself in whatever you are doing in the moment.

7. **Let go of perfectionism.** When you catch yourself judging yourself, learn to dis-engage and simply observe like a little movie. As the Sufi saying goes, "be in the world, but not of it."

Online Resources for Practicing Mindfulness

Largest free on-line library of meditations, courses
https://insighttimer.com

On self-compassion and healing old wounds:
https://www.tarabrach.com/rain-practice-radical-compassion/

https://self-compassion.org

On pain management - mindfulness-based stress reduction (free online course) https://palousemindfulness.com

Mental health resources such as mindfulness, self-compassion, & positive emotions: https://www.rickhanson.net

FOURTH GRACE

Awakening Joy
through Simplicity and Humor

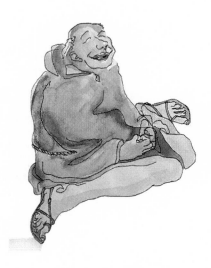

"Angels fly because they take themselves lightly."
—C. K. Chesterton

"In the point of rest at the center of our being, we encounter a world where all things are at rest in the same way. Then a tree becomes a mystery, a cloud a revelation, each man a cosmos of whose riches we can only catch glimpses. The life of simplicity is simple, but it opens to us a book in which we never get beyond the first syllable."
—Dag Hammarskjöld

"It is not the young man who should be considered fortunate but the old man who has lived well, because the young man in his prime wanders much by chance, vacillating in his beliefs, while the old man has docked in the harbor, having safeguarded his true happiness."
—Vatican sayings, 19th c.

"Everyone thinks that his things are not like all the things in the world. And that is why everyone keeps them."
—Antonio Porchia from *Voices*

"Humor extends the shelf life of our sanity."
—Anonymous

"(Humor) keeps (the elderly) rolling, singing a song. When you laugh it's an involuntary explosion of the lungs. The lungs need to replenish themselves with oxygen. So you laugh, you breathe, the blood runs, and everything is circulating. If you don't laugh, you'll die!"
—Mel Brooks

DANIEL KLEIN
AGE 81

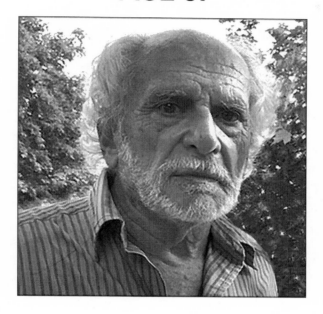

Daniel Klein is an author, philosopher, and great teller of jokes. He studied philosophy at Harvard and went on the become a writer because, in his words, "I do not like to work." He has written for over 40 years and still loves to write. His recent book, Travels with Epicurus is, in essence, a lyrical exploration of his own aging. He describes his late in life journey to Hydra, Greece, where the bounty of a simple life, tied in with the philosophy of Epicurus, led him to pose the question, what does a happy life entail? Which pleasures gratify and endure, and which pleasures are transitory or even lead to pain?

"Nothing is enough for the man to whom enough is too little," he quotes from Epicurus. Dan's journey to Greece led him to believe that adherence to the simplicity of life, making plenty of time for meaningful relationships, and never losing humor are the enduring takeaways that offer a compass in life.

Dan's great passion, of course, is writing. He says that wanting to write "it," the one big success, is one of those pleasures that leads to pain. He has learned to enjoy the process of writing without setting out for the big goal. He's written some of his books with his best friend, with whom he shares a common philosophy of living authentically and who, more importantly, has a delicious sense of humor.

Dan is married and has a daughter and granddaughter, the apples of his eye, but it is equally important for him to balance a good family life with engaging in "'individual" social activities. He remembers his parents, particularly his father, isolated without a network of friends, and vowed early never to repeat this.

How does Dan stay young in his eighties? He says that his creative endeavors keep him focused on the moment where death does not exist. Above all, he sees humor as a source of joy and lightness. Sex and death provoke most anxieties, he reminds, that's why so many jokes are about sex and death, he says. Humor counteracts worries and dread.

"I live on jokes," Dan Klein said. "There's transcendence in humor."

Our American culture strives for perfection—
the perfect house, the perfect body, the perfect job,
the perfect partner. We want to have it all, to do it
all, to be the best. We accumulate stuff we don't need.
We consume more information than we can possibly
process. We damage our bodies with crash diets, Botox,
and plastic surgery to defy our age. We often work too
long and too hard at work we don't enjoy in a culture
that craves and serves winning, success, and money.

This reminds me of the old saying, "He who dies
with the most toys wins." When we value ourselves by
what we can attain rather than simply being who we
are, some is never enough. We always come up short.
Rather than creating and sustaining a simple life that
suits our nature and our values, we complicate our
lives and perpetuate a mindset of scarcity. And, more
often than not, our striving and acquiring create only
temporary satisfaction.

My old friend and client, Pathfinder Betty
MacDonald, long ago learned that things do not buy
happiness. An actor for many years with a passion for
psychodrama, Betty says unabashedly, "I love getting
older. I love slowing down. I've let go of expectations. I
can simply be, happy or not." When we last spoke, she
mused, "It makes me laugh and relax when I realize
that we're just specks of dust on a piece of dung flying
through the universe." Betty is at work on a book about
the joys of aging.

Decluttering Creates Simplicity

In *The Gentle Art of Swedish Death Cleaning*, author Margaret Magnusson, a Swedish woman who tells us she is between 80 and 100 years old, but doesn't reveal her exact age, guides the interested reader to simplify the lives of our forebears by cleaning up our own act while we can and, in so doing, create a simpler, more balanced, and enjoyable daily life for ourselves now and for our loved ones later. Magnusson helps us begin by reminding us. "Do not ever imagine that anyone will wish—or be able—to schedule time off to take care of what you didn't bother to take care of yourself. No matter how much they love you, don't leave this burden to them."

Only six months ago, when we moved from our home of 25 years to our new house, I went through the sorting we all do when downsizing. It was exhausting but felt wonderfully liberating.

The manager of the moving team mentioned a recent client who never threw anything away. She had been renting a locker filled with her old furniture and precious stuff for over 30 years at a cost of hundreds of dollars each month. When he asked her whether her children wanted any of it, she said, " I certainly hope so!"

Nonetheless, death cleaning does not mean that you eliminate your beloved objects, those that make your life comfortable and pleasant, but rather to let go of those things that simply don't reflect who you are or that no longer please you. Magnusson can be quite specific in her advice, suggesting we begin our death cleaning by turning to the largest items—to create space and allow us to reorganize—and turn to our mementos, such as photographs, old letters, and personal papers, last. These can evoke memories and even nostalgia. We must be careful when we give ourselves the time and attention to attend to these special things, that we do not lean toward sentimentality.

Magnusson reminds us that even the most important collection of things carries little weight to others when we're gone. She drives this home with humor by advising, "There's no sense in saving things that will upset your family after you are gone. Save your favorite dildo—but throw away the other 15!"

All in all, death cleaning or decluttering fosters simplicity and ease. My old friend Pathfinder Sarnie Ogus, 93, used to live in a grand Upper East Side apartment in Manhattan. She now relishes her small, Zen-like abode that reflects her sense of inner peace and provides a safe haven from the worrisome world. Sarnie claims that it was a bit difficult at first to let go of some personal items, but it quickly turned into a joyous experience. "It was just so liberating to let go and allow space to open inside of me, as well as on the outside," she said, which reminded me of this story:

In the last century, a tourist from the United States visited the famous Polish rabbi Hafez Hayyim.

He was astonished to see that the rabbi's home was only a simple room filled with books. The only furniture was a table and a bench.

"Rabbi, where is your furniture?" asked the tourist.

"Where's yours?" replied Hafez.

"Mine? But I'm only a visitor here."

"So am I," said the rabbi.

Simple Pleasure as the True Sustenance of Life

The philosopher Epicurus felt that the very purpose of philosophy was to attain a peaceful, joyful life, free from fear and filled with pleasure. Epicurus himself would have loved the following ancient Mulla Nasreddin story:

Nasreddin was eating a poor man's diet of chickpeas and bread. His neighbor, who also claimed to be a wise man was living in a grand house and dining on sumptuous meals provided by the emperor himself. His neighbor told Nasreddin, "if only you would learn to flatter the emperor and be subservient like I do, you would not have to live on chickpeas and bread." Nasreddin replied, "and if only you would learn to love chickpeas and bread, like I do, you would not have to flatter and live subservient to the emperor!"

He championed that simple pleasures are the true sustenance of life, quite in contrast to our Western way intent on striving, the stamp of an overtly patriarchal culture, where accomplishment and power trump love and joy.

Pathfinder Dan Klein sheds light on the bounty of the simple, pleasure-filled life by also suggesting that Epicurean philosophy only began with this notion. It spawns some tough questions, like "what is a happy life?" "which pleasures both gratify and endure?" or "which pleasures are transitory and lead to pain?"

He offers one answer from Epicurus that he agrees with, that is, a happy life is free from the commercial world, quoting the philosopher himself, "Nothing is enough for the man to whom enough is too little." He also notes that Epicurus believed man should free himself "from the prison of everyday affairs and politics," with which Klein disagrees. In keeping with his belief that a person must be true to himself or herself to be happy, he shares that in the current political climate, he feels enlivened by debate and opinion. I tend to agree with him.

A philosopher in his own right, Dan is also a man who's always ready to hear a good joke—and we have shared many during our time together. I laugh out loud when I remember Dan asking: "You know the story about the guy who's our age, in his seventies?" I shook my head.

*"He's walking along and sees a frog. The frog says,
"Old man, pick me up; kiss me; I'll turn into a
beautiful princess and we'll have sex all night." He
picks her up and puts her in his pocket. He keeps
walking along, until she pops out her head and says,
"Old man, didn't you hear me? If you kiss me I'll turn
into a beautiful princess and we'll have sex all night!"
He looks at her and says, "I heard you, Froggie.
Thanks, but honestly, at my age, I'd rather have a
talking frog."*

Laughter and Delight as the Best Medicines

When I interviewed Dr. Irving Milberg, he
mentioned that laughing kept him young. With a
twinkle in her eye my client, Iris Alster said, "If you can
laugh at yourself, life is easy."

When I was in India with my spiritual teacher in
the 1970s, he would advise that seriousness is a disease
that takes an individual out of the current moment.
He taught that such a state of solemnity indicated
one's thinking about the past or imagining possible
or probable futures. When we laugh, we're here now,
in the life we're living. We relish the moment. We
are self-aware; we witness our responses and feelings
but without taking ourselves too seriously. I learned
many years ago from my teacher that seriousness
only exists in the past or the future, while spontaneity
and playfulness, known as *leela* in Sanskrit, live in the

moment. In India, to look through the lens of *leela* is to find enlightenment! We live the essence of life itself. We come alive!

Of course, being serious has its place, such as when studying, rehearsing, analyzing, speculating, and the like, but even then, it does us well to not take ourselves too seriously, to lighten our load with humor.

Two memories come to mind from my own experience. The first occurred when I was in my late twenties, attending a ten-day meditation camp in the mountains and jungles of Rajasthan, India. My spiritual teacher was teaching in an old castle on Mount Abu, considered a holy mountain. We practiced meditation at set times of the day and listened to his discourses at other set times. We rose at 5:30 a.m. each day for the first meditation. It was quite cold early in the morning, barely above freezing, though reaching a comfortable 70 during the day. The first meditation was called the Laughing meditation. We were asked to begin our day by laughing out loud, even if forced when we started. Though we hated to leave our warm beds after the prior full day of meditation and discourses, we began the day with, "HA HA!" Many of the attendees rented rooms from people who lived in houses on the mountain. We could all hear each other's "HA HAs" through one house to another until the whole mountain came alive with contagious laughter. These days beginning with laughter created a levity that lasted all day long.

Laughter naturally discards the excess, the debris, and changes everything.

The second memory comes from a weekend workshop that I attended where the British philosopher and writer Alan Watts presided. I clearly remember him walking about the campus spouting, "HA, HA, HA!" When I asked him what he was doing, he told me he was developing his belly laugh. It's not surprising that Watts once said, "Real religion is the transformation of anxiety into laughter." He also remarked, "…If this state of consciousness (presence to the universal mystery of existence) could become more universal, the pretentious nonsense, which passes for serious business of the world, would dissolve in laughter," pertinent guidance for the current unsettling state of the world's affairs.

The teachings of modern and ancient mystics alike declare that our laughter originates from the very source of our being.

In *Healthy at 100*, author John Robbins notes that the elders—in all four of the cultures he cites as living long, healthy lives—exhibited relentless senses of humor. Though often poor, humor and levity nourished and sustained them.

Robbins also shares what a friend told him about his experiences with the Bushmen of Southern Africa, "When I was there, I would sit out every night close to their huts and listen to the joy in their conversations and laughter. It is remarkable how much happiness they experience in their everyday life...the unconditional love that they have for one another and for all life is a model for the rest of the world to follow." If only it could be so!

Political journalist, professor, and peace advocate Norman Cousins, who wrote *The Anatomy of an Illness*, was a most enthusiastic and informed patient, believing and proving that a positive attitude with a good sense of humor could heal the best of us. Suffering from a debilitating, incurable connective-tissue disease, he shares how, while in hospital planning "his escape" to a hotel to better recover, he experimented with creating laughter as a biological antidote to pain. He firmly believed that affirmative emotions enhanced body chemistry and he intended to prove it. Starting with amusing movies, Allen Funt, host of the TV show "Candid Camera," sent Cousins the classic episodes along with a movie projector. Next he got access to some old Marx Brothers films.

Cousins relays his joyous discovery that ten minutes of belly laughter gave him over two hours of anesthetic relief for pain-free sleep. (He felt excruciating pain in his spine and joints.) While recovering, he used the projector, with his nurse's help, at intervals of pain onset, to watch a humorous film, such as his beloved Marx Brothers. He believed that if the pain had subsided with his laughter, the inflammation that caused it would likely diminish as well. He was elated to find a physiologic basis for the ancient theory that laughter is good medicine.

My own great-grandmother, a healer and a Sephardic Jew in pre-WWII Greece, known in her village as "the little doctor," told Mulla Nasreddin stories to her "patients." Nasreddin's tales were usually humorous stories but the lessons were serious, made palpable and memorable by their satirical edge.

The following Nasreddin story speaks to the age-old tendency to look for the key to freedom, love, fulfillment, and meaning in the light, where one believes they can see clearly, rather than all too often in the darker places, where the key has likely been lost:

> *A man is walking home late one night when he sees an anxious Mulla Nasreddin down on all fours, crawling on his hands and knees on the road, searching frantically under a streetlight for something on the ground.*
>
> *"Mulla, what have you lost?" the passerby asks. "I am searching for my key," Nasreddin says worriedly. "I'll help you look," the man says and joins Mulla Nasreddin in the search. Soon both men are down on their knees under the streetlight, looking for the lost key. After some time, the man asks Nasreddin, "Tell me, Mulla, do you remember where exactly you dropped the key?" Nasreddin waves his arm back toward the darkness and says, "Over there, in my*

house. I lost the key inside my house..." Shocked and *exasperated, the passerby jumps up and shouts at Mulla Nasreddin, "Then why are you searching for the key out here in the street?" "Because there is more light here than inside my house," Mulla Nasreddin answers nonchalantly.*

In Western society, when we retire from a job held for many years, we have time at last for more intelligent play. It doesn't mean that we take life any less seriously. It means that our life becomes more fluid, more spontaneous, and likely more fun. We might say life has more soul, more joy. We can even laugh at ourselves!

Cultivating the Seeds of the Fourth Grace: Awakening Joy through Simplicity and Humor

1. **Declutter and let go.** Margaret Magnussun's wonderful book *The Gentle Art of Swedish Death Cleaning: How to Free Yourself and Your Family from a Lifetime Clutter* sets us straight about what to keep and what not to. Her rule is simple: *If it brings you pleasure, keep it; if there's "should" in your decision, let the thing go.*

2. **Slow down to "smell the roses."** Moving slower brings grace, awareness, and opens our senses to the present.

3. **There's nowhere to go, you're there.** Life is not a series of goal setting, meeting, or failing;

115

true meaning is not over there but wherever, whenever we are aware and present in our life.

4. **Let's play!** Usually we are so busy reaching our destination or goal that we forget to enjoy the process. Just having fun can assuage boredom and lighten a heavy heart. Like play, creativity invites us to lose ourselves, to be open to surprise, to leap into the realm of the imagination. We might ask, "Does play bring joy or does our joy inform our play?"

5. **Practice laughing and smiling.** Tell more jokes and watch funny movies. Here's a good meditation for first awakening in the morning: Before opening your eyes, think of a humorous event or movie that made you smile and giggle inside. When the smile on your face becomes real, it's time to get off to a good start of your day. Remember to smile at yourself, when you pass a mirror. It will lift your mood.

6. **Play music** that makes you feel good.

7. **Turn off the news.** Be informed, not obsessed!

Online Resources for Awakening Joy through Simplicity and Humor

Laugh Therapy:

http://www.laughteryogaonthephone.com/laughter-yoga-on-the-phone-1.html

FIFTH GRACE

Pursuing Your Passion:
clarifying a long-dreamed vision or unrealized idea and practicing it

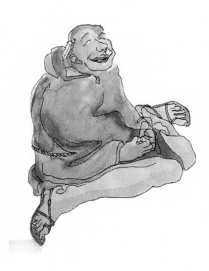

"People like you and I, though mortal, of course, like everyone else, do not grow old no matter how long they live. We never cease to stand like curious children before the great mystery into which we were born."
—Albert Einstein

"My body is on the earth, but my head is in the stars."
—Maude (Ruth Gordon)
in the film *Harold and Maude*

"The bird doesn't sing because it has an answer. It sings because it has a song."
—Maya Angelou

"They will say that you are on the wrong road, if it is your own."
—Antonio Porchia from *Voices*

"No one is so old as those who have outlived their enthusiasm."
—Henry David Thoreau

"There is no cure for birth and death, but to enjoy the interval"
—George Santayana

"Don't retire…never retire. Ever!!"
—Pathfinder David Lewine

GILLIAN JAGGER
AGE 87

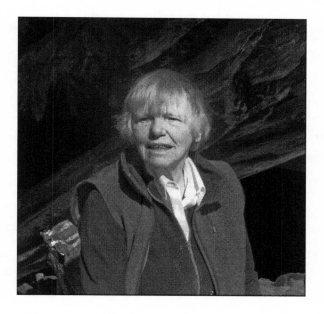

Fifteen years ago I had the great honor to meet
Gillian Jagger, *an artist and sculptor of world renown.*
She consulted me because of excruciating pain in both of her
knees, and knee replacement had been recommended. Gillian
was afraid of surgery and committed herself to trying an
alternative route first. It turned out that acupuncture and
herbal remedies alleviated her pain, and she never went
under the knife. She became a regular client and allowed me
to help her with both physical and psychological issues.

Gillian was brought up in England by a beautiful but
emotionally disturbed mother who was driven by paranoia
and jealousy. In a psychotic episode, her mother had even

attempted to strangle Gillian, and the child had barely escaped. Thankfully, her father showered his daughter with affection and love, encouraging her to believe in herself. Charles Sargeant Jagger was a famous sculptor in England, known to this day for his war monuments. Gillian vividly remembers his passion for creating.

Tragically, Gillian lost her father when he was only 48 and she, only five. Soon afterward, her older sister, who had been great comfort to her, also died. A protective and affectionate German nanny left the family soon after. With World War II coming, her mother took Gillian out of boarding school, a safe haven, and relocated to the United States. Her mother's hostility and unpredictability had only gotten worse. Gillian endured tirades of blame and criticism during which her mother told her that she would amount to nothing, ridiculing her for wanting to be an artist.

But, Gillian felt a growing desire to create, as her father had done. She enrolled herself in art school, and a prolific career unfolded. She became known for her innovative style in the New York City art community, but she consistently refused labeling of any kind. She insisted on doing what came spontaneously through her, rather than overthinking her process.

Through her art, Gillian transcended the multiple traumas that she had survived. Her deep connection with her father's passion for art had become her guiding force in life, translating into a burning, lifelong need to create.

Recently, after our interview for this book, Gillian took a fall that partially paralyzed her. No longer able to sculpt or paint, she took to writing by dictation, continuing to insist on channeling her creative spirit. She died in November 2019.

DAVID LEWINE
——— AGE 86 ———

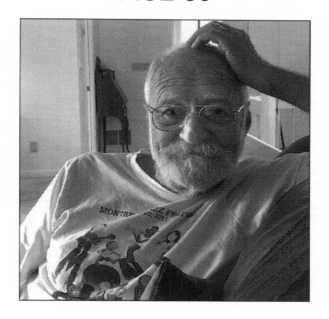

David Lewine *grew up in a poor neighborhood within a family of discord, plagued by a lack of discipline and palpable unhappiness. He was a troubled youth who constantly got into conflicts, small and large. He graduated from high school with difficulties and worked odd jobs for*

a while. When he finally had a streak of luck and success by becoming foreman of a construction team, he messed up his chances and got arrested for driving while intoxicated.

David realized that he needed structure in his life. He enrolled in the Marine Corps and stayed there for many years during which time he got married and had five children. After his honorable discharge, he moved his family to New York in order to work for his father's insurance company, in spite of his poor relationship with his father and intense dislike for this line of work. David tried hard to earn a decent living for his family, but he was not cut out for this kind of life, and he fell into a deep depression.

Music saved him. He bought a guitar and taught himself to play. It didn't take long for him to become obsessed and this time he did become successful, which set him on a new course. He was making a good living as a music teacher and was consumed by this new passion. Later, he picked up photography, which also provided him a good income.

In 1984, David's marriage ended, and he became estranged from his children. Alone, David searched for a deeper meaning in his life. He stumbled upon yoga, which was not yet popular in the United States. He felt that yoga provided him with a physical discipline and instilled in him a sense of existential meaning. In search of spirituality, he set out to study yoga with masters in the United States and later India. Meditation and yoga become his life and he immersed himself in it.

Back in the United States, David believed his mission was to give back the wealth of knowledge he had gained. He started teaching yoga in schools, organized yoga classes and meditation gatherings, often without reimbursement .

Today he does "karma yoga," (giving-back yoga) at a veterans' hospital where he teaches and assists fellow veterans.

Finding his passions helped David survive a job he hated, a deep depression, and the separation from his family. Through living a spiritual life with passion, he found his present wife, a woman he had known for 26 years, who shares his joy of giving back.

When you are passionate about your life, you may enjoy many creative activities, such as gardening, cooking, painting, or carpentry, or you may have one primary focus, such as mastering a musical instrument or writing a book. The stage of life designated in Western culture as "retirement" opens time to explore these things, to not only have more fun, but also to re-create your life, to make it new!

A passion is an intense feeling. Our passion awakens when we resonate with another person; this type of passion can be sexual or romantic in nature. Or our passion can be ignited by engaging in a creative activity, such as playing the guitar, singing in a chorus, writing poetry, painting, woodworking, or maintaining and sailing a boat.

I like how the *Urban Dictionary* defines the second type of passion: "Passion is when you put more energy into something than is required to do it. It is more than just enthusiasm or excitement; passion is ambition that is materialized into action to put as much heart, mind, body, and soul into something as is possible."

When we allow ourselves to be consumed by such a passion, we enter what psychologist Daniel Goleman calls a state of "flow." When we're in flow, the constraints of time and place become irrelevant because we're caught up in a process that brings us pure, unmitigated joy.

My own passions inspired me to write this book. These include my love of reading, learning, the beauty I capture through photography, and, of course, holistic healing.

When I was young and carefree, I would drive cross-country with a friend. In each region that we passed through, whether mountains or desert or farmland, I would press one or more of my fingers down on my flute and allow the currents of air, the wind, to play my instrument. Each landscape emitted a unique sonorous quality, evoking a resonant chord or song. Did the wind resonate with the instrument or the instrument with the wind? It didn't matter; the moment held the meaning of the sound. Though I wouldn't have known how to put it into words back then, in those moments I was in a state of flow.

When we step into this "cosmic" current and resonate with the life force, we might say, we enter "the zone." Some say that a divine spark urges us to create, to tap into our own unique creative process. Whatever ignites that creative spark in you, whether learning a craft, traveling, gardening, cooking—you name it!— pursuing a passion can infuse life with meaning. In fact, it can become your life's purpose. As so many of us today in the wake of COVID 19, my son, a musician living in Denver, is managing his isolation. When fear and stress become overwhelming, he told me he picks up his guitar and plays or composes music. This allows him to enter the "flow," and helps to transform his fear into a creative force. It's one of those obscure gifts that this pandemic may be gifting us!

The secular culture might say that spirit sparks our passion in life, the spirit that moves us and brings us most alive. Each of the Pathfinders in this book has shared as much, even if they are not overtly spiritually minded people. Each has said in one way or another that when tapped into a true passion, he or she embodies the passion itself.

For instance, when Sir Winston Churchill gave up the statesmanship phase of his life, he turned toward his passion for painting. He even wrote a book in his final years, *Painting as a Pastime*, about the spiritual depth he experienced through painting. In it, he quotes an American psychologist: "Worry is a spasm of the emotion; the mind catches hold of something and will not let it go." Churchill adds, "It is useless to argue with the mind in this condition. The stronger the will, the more futile the task. One can only gently insinuate something else into its convulsive grasp. And if this something is rightly chosen, if it is really attended by the illumination of another field of interest, gradually, and often quite swiftly, the old undue grip relaxes, and the process of recuperation and repair begins."

Think of Benjamin Franklin who lived to be 84, even though the life expectancy of a man in Colonial America was only 33 years. Franklin lived a life of purpose as printer, publisher, author, humorist, statesman, scientist, inventor, innovator, ambassador, and, of course, a signer of the Declaration of Independence.

In his memoir *It Takes a Long Time to Become Young* (the title of which was taken from a quote by Picasso) the actor, writer, and director Garson Kanin recalled being asked frequently by admirers to reveal the secret behind his wife, the actress Ruth Gordon's, boundless energy and enthusiasm for life, which kept her bright-eyed, perky, and pursuing her craft well into her eighties. Gordon, who was also a screenwriter and playwright, is perhaps best known for her lively performance as an 80-year-old woman having a love affair with a 20-year-old man in the cult classic movie *Harold and Maude*. Kanin declares that there was no secret to his beloved spouse's vitality but rather a sheer "desire to work, to create, to stay in action…" Gordon's appreciation for life in all its complexity and simplicity offered her endless opportunities for discovery. She believed that nothing was more important than imagination and endurance.

This reminds me of a favorite story:

[There was] a man who died and found himself in a beautiful place, surrounded by every conceivable comfort. A white-jacketed man came to him and said, "You may have anything you choose—any food, any pleasure, any kind of entertainment.

The man was delighted, and for days he sampled all the delicacies and experiences of which he had only dreamed of on earth. But one day he grew bored with all of it, and calling the attendant to him, he said, "I'm tired of all this. I need something to do. What kind of work can you give me?"

The attendant sadly shook his head and replied, "I'm sorry sir. That's the one thing we can't do for you. There is no work here for you."

To which the man answered, "That's a fine thing. I might as well be in hell."

The attendant said softly, "Where do you think you are, sir?"

—From *Stories of the Spirit, Stories of the Heart*, edited by Christina Feldman and Jack Kornfield

Creativity Late in Life

I believe that like good wine our creativity finds its full bouquet with age. In our later years, our creative energies are free to expand. After many years of learning the mechanics of our art, we can synthesize and practice our knowledge, giving it our full, unique expression.

Many people have created works of lasting beauty and importance in their elder years. Buckminster Fuller continued to generate new ideas at 80. Henri Matisse, Pablo Picasso, Mary Cassatt, Michelangelo, and Leonardo Da Vinci all became more artistically creative as they aged. Grandma Moses did not even begin her artwork until she was 72. And, Georgia O'Keeffe painted daily into her nineties. The spaciousness of life often eases our thinking mind, allowing for deeper intuitive awareness that can create new ideas, open to unimpeded inspiration, solve problems, and make better decisions. [20]

If you're entering or well into your aging years, and tapping again or anew into your creative energies, you're in good company!

---

[20] Zalman Schachter-Shalomi and Ronald S. Miller, *From Age-ing to Sage-ing: A Revolutionary Approach to Growing Older* (New York: Grand Central Publishing, 2014), p. 43-44

Elder Creative Luminaries

- At 90, **Marc Chagall** said, "I work as long as I have the strength. Without my work, my life would be idiotic." Tapping his temple, he said, "Even when I'm not working, I'm working."

- The architect **Frank Lloyd Wright**'s final work was even more imaginative and innovative than his earlier concepts.

- **Carl Reiner**, who laughed his way into old age, and wrote four books well into his 90s.

- **Sigmund Freud**, the founder of psychoanalysis, continued to write, research, and study until his death at 83.

- **Clara Barton**, founder of the Red Cross, at 90, worked 14 hours each day. "While the strength is given me," she declared, "I have no right to lay it down."

- **Albert Einstein**, the greatest scientist of the 20th century, continued his work until the end, declaring from his deathbed at age 76, "I want to go when I want. It is tasteless to prolong life artificially. I have done my share; it is time to go."

- **Thomas Edison**, the pioneering American inventor, is believed to have had a third peak in creative productivity between ages 70 and 75, remaining active until his death at 83.

> And many elders still living continue to thrive, such as:
>
> - **At 98, Norman Lear** is still making us laugh.
> - **Shirley MacLaine, 86,** and **Betty White, 98,** still perform!
> - **Noam Chomsky**, the renowned linguist and social critic, is 91 and still writing and teaching.
> - **Jane Goodall**, the pioneering British anthropologist and primatologist is 86.
> - **Jane Fonda**, 82, is still going full force as an actress and a social activist.
>
> And, we only recently lost the inimitable U.S. Supreme Court Justice **Ruth Bader Ginsburg** at 87.

A complete listing of creative luminaries who continued working well into old age would fill an entire book.

Artist and sculptor Gillian Jagger noted, when we spoke, that much later in life, when she returned to a previously conceived piece, she was struck by how her concept of that piece had grown. "I never would have thought that as I got older, I could expand my work," she confided. "Now, I begin to think that we all need to keep life fresh. Even though I no longer need the physical stimulation, let's say, of riding a horse, I must keep going. My art goes along with me, wherever I go. It's the thing that inspires me."

Jagger shared this message, I believe, to encourage all older creative folks: "I believe in living an optimal experience while you can. Be open to your instincts. Don't allow yourself to be labeled by others or through the media. The later years offer a renewal or rebirth, where we must expand our intuition. Always remain open to possibility rather than falling prey to depression or just plain giving up because you believe you are too old to create or follow a passion."

None of the individuals I've mentioned had any desire to retire. All the Pathfinders consider their creative process a necessity to their very being. Their endeavors are not guided by the intention to create a product. Rather, they are a response to an internal urge to act in keeping with one's inner core. Such people, I believe, age naturally and most gracefully.

Even those who have passed on since our interviews continued to do what they loved to do, as long as they could, as long as they lived.

Such dedication applies to any true vocation or avocation that carries the soul's calling. Religious and spiritual people, or, for example, hospice workers and others in the helping professions, through their work in the service of others, tap into a creative source, something larger than themselves beyond ego. People who are able to connect to the generative flow of their existence feel part of a meaningful whole in contrast to those who feel useless because they don't know what to do with their lives after they retire.

In an interview, the celebrated Russian composer, pianist and conductor Igor Stravinsky, then in his eighties, was asked if it was more difficult to find inspiration as a composer in old age. He smiled, saying that the reporters were looking at him as an old man, but that he didn't experience himself that way. So the question had no meaning for him. [21]

Stravinsky's remark is sound advice for any older person. Ignore another's limiting view, which may perceive you as older than you sense you are. We must be true to our soul's age, not our age in numbers or as indicated by poor health. These are meaningless to the soul. It would do us all well to heed Stravinsky's response when asked if his old age impacted his inspiration: "I don't know what it means to be old."

I love what Sam Ulano, "Mr. Rhythm," a notorious drummer and drum teacher, shared, at 85, in his soulful book *Keep Swinging: Approach Your Senior Years without Skipping a Beat.* He says: "Liking what you do, to me, is not sufficient. I want to do only what I love. This way I can work day after day at my inner joy....I have many friends who just spend day after day searching for that one thing that would give them the inner glow that comes from doing what you love to do. It's not easy to

---

[21] Thomas Moore. *Ageless Soul: The Lifelong Journey Toward Meaning and Joy* (New York: St. Martin's Press, 2017) p. 46

find, but it's there and when we recognize it, we know we've found our greatest desire."

Yvonne Pastolove, 84, the mother of a dear friend, began writing historical novels at age 80, after her husband died. Yvonne's writing totally absorbs her. She says that research in particular "exercises" her brain, keeping her vital, curious, and engaged. During our interview, when the topic of her writing came up, she glowed. We both understood that she had tapped into her flow, her creative source. She is now on her fourth novel.

Then there are people like Pathfinder Iris Alster, who find sheer delight in simply being alive. When asked to name her passion, Iris exclaimed, "People are my passion—people and my joy for living." Iris loves to travel. She told me this memorable story about her trip to Tibet.

> *"Tibet had always fascinated me. We travelled in trucks on rutted road; we relieved ourselves in holes in the ground and bathed in streams. To get to one monastery we had to travel by boat from the ship. The oil in the monastery smelled horrid back then before they began to use ghee...*
>
> *All of a sudden, a young female Tibetan leader came and called out for us to come. I thought there must be a fire but there wasn't, rather a gathering of monks who were preparing to chant, the young apprentices*

pouring tea for them. Then, came the instruments—cymbals and long horns. It was just marvelous! There were eight of us on that trip of every religion. I was the only Jew. All of a sudden, the chant became haunting, captivating each and every one of us, moving us to the core. We each knew then and there that there was but one God. We all were moved to tears, the men as well as the women. It was a true epiphany for each of us."

Iris didn't say so, but I believe that experience changed her life. More recently, at age 94, she travelled to Southeast Asia, downriver to Myanmar.

And, there's my friend and client Carolee Schneemann, an American visual artist, renowned for her provocative artistic commentaries on the female body, sexuality and gender. Carolee's distinctly feminist vision aimed to thwart the patriarchal disconnect between woman as individual and woman as artist; through her multimedia artwork, she celebrated sexual expression and liberation. Carolee believed that her passion for making art and her commitment to social justice fostered her longevity. We lost her in March 2019.

Suffering as the Alchemist's Flame

Up until now we've considered passion and creativity as flow, a connection with Source that lives through us as a creative passion. This energy can also make itself known through pain and suffering, which forces us to look within. Within this internal space, often melancholy, we must have the courage to wait and to trust that a deep awareness wants to express itself. For example, suffering has inspired some of our most memorable poetry, music, and song.

Alchemy is the art of turning base metal into gold. In the philosophical, even mystical sense, alchemy can refine and transform a muddled consciousness into clear consciousness. And pain and/or suffering often initiate such a transformation. Pain and/or suffering are the catalytic agents, the alchemist's flames. We must remember, too, that alchemy cannot occur unless a vessel is securely closed. Metaphorically this refers to an individual's ability to embrace and withstand discomfort in service to birthing a creative vision or necessary healing, such as through abstention from addictive behavior.

In the depth of depression, Pathfinder David Lewine discovered the guitar. Playing it became an intense passion that became an obsession. He claims to have played up to 14 hours a day, able to "disappear" into the music, feeling renewed with joy. Living this passion led him to the study of yoga and meditation. David's experience shows how passion nourishes itself, reflecting the Buddhist concept that "Suffering opens the path to joy."

Pathfinder Gillian Jagger grew up through a childhood of despair. Her father, to whom she felt deeply connected, died when she was very young and her mother blamed Gillian for his death. Her pain and fear forced young Gillian to seek refuge in nature. The artistic girl's refuge became her inspiration.

As the spiritual teacher Ram Dass puts it, suffering can be a form of "fierce grace."

This time of plague invites us to envision the suffering in our own souls and those of others around the world and in our own backyards. Such conscious contemplation fuels the "alchemist's flame," thus creating space for rebirth.

Lewis Richmond reminds us that the Buddhist adage, "all life is suffering," does not mean life is only suffering but that disappointment, loss, and frustration—all manner of difficulty—physical, emotional, or spiritual—is integral to living. As an antidote to suffering, Richmond recommends practicing kindness in all of our encounters, especially with those cycling through the phases of aging.

This teaching story, called "Struggle," illustrates this point.

> *A man found a cocoon of the Emperor moth and took it home to watch it emerge. One day a small opening appeared, and for several hours the moth struggled but couldn't seem to force its body past a certain point. Deciding something was wrong, the man took scissors and snipped the remaining bit of cocoon. The moth*

emerged easily, its body large and swollen, the wings small and shriveled. The man expected that in a few hours the wings would spread out in their natural beauty, but they did not. Instead of developing into a creature free to fly, the moth spent its life dragging around a swollen body and shriveled wings.

The constricting cocoon and the struggle necessary to pass through the tiny opening are God's way of forcing fluid from the body into the wings. The "merciful" snip was, in reality, cruel. Sometimes the struggle is exactly what we need.

In the end, authentic feeling, whether melancholy, inspirational, or even contented, can fuel passion and give meaning to life well into old age, even in the midst of undue challenges.

Cultivating the Seeds of the Fifth Grace: Pursuing Your Passion

1. **If you love it, do it.** Whatever brings you joy will likely also bring you spiritual well-being. What's more, pursuing your passion can help keep you emotionally balanced and mentally and physically fit.

2. **Curiosity can lead to passion.** When you're not sure what turns you on, or if you find yourself drawn to many things and can't decide which direction to follow, try to notice what makes

you the most curious. Staying curious as we grow older awakens new energy and renews latent desires. Curiosity can be a stepping-stone toward your next chapter.

3. **Turn on the tap with mind-body practice.** We're all born with the ability to be creative. Sadly, the challenges we face in adolescence and adulthood may cause us to lose touch with the creative impulse that came effortlessly when we were young children. But there is good news. As we age, we can use mind-body techniques such as relaxation, visualization, and free movement to enliven our intuition and re-activate our natural ability to tap into our creativity.

4. **Explore ways to feed your passion:** Take classes in painting, writing, dancing, or singing. If your passion resonates with helping others in hospitals, contact local community boards, which offer numerous opportunities to identify the volunteering opportunity that can enrich your soul.

5. **Bring joy into whatever you do.** Even if through necessity or circumstance, you must accept your lot, you can find joy when you look for it in whatever you are doing.

6. **If you have trouble connecting to a passion, think of something that excited you when you were young, and reconnect to that feeling.** Does that "thing" still rock your boat, or can you imagine something new and exciting? No filter, let your mind explore.

Online Resources for Pursuing Your Passion:

Any commentary about creativity and aging should include reference to the National Center for Creative Aging, which has been in the forefront of the creative aging movement, through community centers, local collage continuing-education classes, libraries, and museums.

https://creativeaging.org

Finding your passion:

https://www.entrepreneur.com/article/309286

https://blogs.wsj.com/briefly/2014/12/22/how-to-find-your-passion-in-retirement-at-a-glance/

http://www.oprah.com/supersoulsunday/the-secret-to-finding-your-passion-hint-its-not-what-you-think_1

Discovering what you love most is an adventure in itself.

https://www.psychologytoday.com/us/blog/prescriptions-life/201205/five-steps-finding-your-passion

Fun part time jobs:

http://sixtyandme.com/9-fun-part-time-jobs-for-retirees/

SIXTH GRACE

Moving and Being Moved

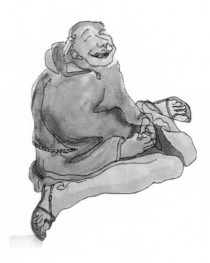

"In the woods I feel that nothing can befall me...which nature cannot repair."
—Ralph Waldo Emerson

"Those who do not find time for exercise will have to find time for illness."
—Edward Stanley, 15th Earl of Derby

"Walking is man's best medicine."
—Hippocrates

"Life is a verb."
—Charlotte Perkins Gillman

"Be not afraid of going slowly; be only afraid of standing still."
—Chinese Proverb

"I especially love to dance and do so at every opportunity!"
— Pathfinder Benedicta Nieves

"I do some sort of exercise everyday—yoga three times each week and walking in nature whenever weather permits."
—Pathfinder Iris Alster

"Not a day goes by when I don't do yoga or exercise."
—Pathfinder David Lewine

SARNIE OGUS
AGE 93

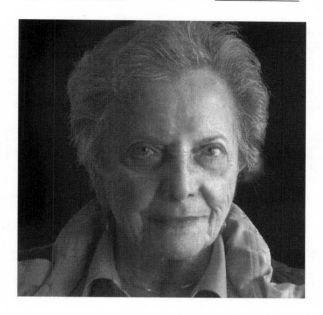

In the 1970s I set out to become a teacher of The Alexander Technique, a form of movement therapy that was created by F. M. Alexander to help people with a variety of physical ailments. One of my teachers at the time was **Sarnie Ogus,** *whose body posture and movement seemed to suggest that, although very grounded, she was perpetually lifting herself into space. She was simply beautiful in her lightness. During the two years of studying with her we became close friends. I eagerly listened to her truly riveting life story and the path that led her to becoming an Alexander teacher.*

Born before the Great Depression, Sarnie witnessed
the decline of her family's financial well-being and
the breakup of her family. As her parents struggled to
build a new existence, she was sent to her oldest sister
in Wisconsin and later to her other sister in California.
Through circuitous routes, she became involved in MGM
Studios in Los Angeles, where she met her husband, a
cinematographer. They had four children and, when he
became more successful, the family moved to New York
City, where they led a glamorous life. She had everything
that her mother had wanted for her. But as her children
became independent, Sarnie felt empty. The realization
that her identity hinged on a privileged life provided
by her husband depressed her. She found the strength to
separate from him and set out on a path to find herself.

After studying dance she began to support herself as
a dance teacher, but a traffic accident interfered with her
newfound passion. In 1969 at 45, a taxi rear-ended her
car, and she was thrown from her seat. Left incapacitated
and living on pain medication, she eventually was
diagnosed with a disc injury, which supposedly warranted
surgery. Looking for alternative methods she found The
Alexander Technique, which saved her from surgery and set
her on her path.

Unfortunately, Sarnie and I lost touch for many years.
When I started to conceive the general idea for this book,
Sarnie came to mind. I contacted her and we immediately
renewed our friendship, as if no time had passed. She

sounded youthful and strong. She told me about some life changes, like simplifying her life, downsizing from a sprawling house into a one-bedroom apartment where she had created a space of sparse beauty for meditation. I was eager to see Sarnie and her surrounds.

When I met her in person I was impressed but not surprised to see a woman appearing much younger than her age. She has maintained her grace, buoyancy, and beautifully elongated posture, yet appears grounded and purposeful in her movements. Her enthusiasm for life, for meditation, and for cultural nurturance are unchanged after 45 years. The living space she had created reflected what she was all about: the essential lies within. This informs her purpose in life, which radiates serenity and peace. At 95, she continues to teach master classes around the country for The Alexander Technique, continuing to inspire her students to be mindful of their bodies within space and to be an alert witness to each and every moment in time. Sarnie said it best herself: "I am perfectly happy not knowing what the future brings. It's all here now." This sums up her philosophy of aging, "life is just a dance."

When asked to write a book on his longevity and vitality, the comedian Dick Van Dyke, now 94, replied, "It would be a short book; it would simply say, "keep moving!"

Inactivity breeds weariness, boredom, frustration, anxiety, and, in time, irritability, and bad temper. When we keep moving, doing the exercise that suits our body and our mind, we prevent stagnation. Getting stuck mentally, emotionally, or spiritually interrupts one's natural flow. In essence, stagnation breeds disease.

Gerontologists agree that to stay young the human being must stay active. The elixir of life is not only physical activity but also mental stimulation. As Bob Dylan said, "He who's not busy being born, is busy dying!" We need to avoid mental ruts, fixed habits, old and intractable ways of functioning, which stimulate our decline. Movement, which includes learning and growth, keeps us young. Learn a language or a manual skill, ride a bike, take up a musical instrument, try voice lessons, and so on. When you keep your synapses firing, you develop new neurons!

Remember, we are always in a continual state of becoming. As Ray Kroc, the founder of McDonald's once said, "When you're green you grow; when you're ripe you rot." Stagnation kills us—physically, emotionally, mentally, and spiritually. Awakening to this awareness is the first step toward changing it and creating generative life patterns.

Moving as Essential to the Flow of Life

I explain this diagnostic concept with this important wisdom: never drink from a stagnant pool; only drink from the stream where water flows freely. We all know that blocked water pools, thus providing a breeding ground for pathogens to congregate and pollute. By moving away the twigs and debris, which block the movement of water, flow continues and re-creates health.

The same concept applies to acupuncture/ acupressure when we press or needle certain points on the body, which intends to unblock stagnation and ensure "flow." Dis-ease is simply that, an interruption in flow.

All of Traditional Chinese medicine is based on the fundamental principle that movement is essential to the flow of life. Stasis can, of course, occur from the outside in, such as through accidents, operations, falls or even adverse climatic factors, but stasis can also emerge from within through emotional and/or spiritual impact, such as unexpressed anger, prolonged fear, grief, or even incessant worry.

The acupuncturist's function is to resolve blockage and re-establish "flow" of energy. In life, we endeavor shed light on those places, physical and emotional, where we feel stuck, and imagine ways to recreate flow.

Chungliang Al Huang was a Tai Chi master with whom I studied during my three summers at the Esalen Institute. We would practice the form each morning on the deck overlooking the cliffs of Big Sur. He fully embodied the Tai Chi form, in accordance with the Tao. He taught his students how to connect with the vital current, to feel the force (chi) moving through our bodies and to guide it, allowing the form to manifest through each of us. Rather than learn the movements by heart, he encouraged us to truly feel how each manifested within and through us.

For thousands of years and continuing to this very day, millions and millions of people in all parts of China gather together in parks and halls to practice the ancient art of Tai Chi, a series of movements that are meant to connect its participants to the vital "chi" energy and to move it through the body via the channels, which nourish and support the functioning of all bodily organs. According to Tai Chi philosophy, the life force, our chi, moves through us, thus connecting heaven and earth. We become the bridge. Many studies today affirm the health and longevity benefits of Tai Chi, known as the elixir of long life.

During this time of social isolation, I reclaimed my Tai Chi practice, a gift that keeps on giving. It not only keeps my muscles loose and limber, but it deepens my meditation practice each time I practice the form. I thank my friend and Tai Chi teacher Alan Bandes as well as Berit Schumann for helping me to renew my passion for this sublime form.

I recently had the honor of reconnecting with my original Tai Chi master more than 40 years after we first met at the Esalen Institute near Big Sur, California. We spent a day together. At 81, Chungliang was as youthful and vital as ever. Still a conduit for the life force, he dances and does Tai Chi every day. Winking at me, he said that he was jealous of my white hair and balding head, which made me look like a sage. Poor Chungliang has to endure his full head of jet-black hair!

Physical Activity Prolongs Life—Enjoy it!

A gerontologist who had studied the Abkhazian people's longevity in the Russian steppes for many years speculated that their perpetual physical activity enhanced the amount of oxygen supplied to their hearts. This was confirmed when the *Journal of Epidemiology and Community Health* published a study in 2005 that found that those living in mountain terrains live longer than those in the lowlands. Plus, the Abkhazians never become sedentary. Their elders continue to chop wood, haul water, and work in orchards and gardens, all at high altitude. [22]

---

[22] John Robbins, *Healthy at 100: The Scientifically Proven Secrets of the World's Healthiest and Longest-Lived People* (Ballantine Books: New York, 2006) p. 10

Where the Abkhazians daily traverse (and enjoy) their mountainous terrain, as the Vilcabamban people of the Andes Mountains do in Ecuador, the elderly in Hunza in the northernmost tip of Pakistan, live within the fertile valley of a dramatic Himalayan mountain range with peaks as high as 20,000 feet. With sure-footed agility, they nonetheless hike up and down very steep hillsides well into their nineties.

Western life does not require that we climb mountains to work, unless we live in San Francisco, but hectic city life and a slower country living invite a specific kind of exercise—walking in the City and hiking in the country or doing outside chores. To ensure consistency as you grow older, it helps to map your choice of exercise to a practice that you enjoy. This could be yoga, walking, hiking in nature, or many other choices.

Pathfinder Emelina Edwards, 79, found that movement literally saved her life. In her fifties after a nasty divorce, she fell into a severe depression and considered ending her life. She was stuck and stagnant in her despair, as is common in such a state, where one cannot see the light at the end of the tunnel. She suddenly realized that she lived in a body that no one could take away from her. Determined to get healthy, she joined a gym and began to work out each and every day. Not only did she recover, she continues to thrive. See her story at the beginning of the next chapter.

Then there's Tao Porchon-Lynch of Scarsdale, New York, who taught yoga until 100, which she had been practicing since she was a child in India. In a 2016 article in *The New York Times*, the reporter noted her instructions to her class: "Feel your whole body singing out and hold. The ladder of life will take you to your inner self."

After class she continued, "Whatever you put in your mind materializes. Within yourself, there's an energy, but unless you use it, it dissipates. And that's when you get old." She passed peacefully in 2020 at 102 years old.

Ida Keeling, 103, who was interviewed in the documentary, *If You're Not in the Obits, Eat Breakfast,* began running at 65 after a severe depression ensued when her son was killed. To this day, over 35 years later, she continues to run marathons and compete. Ida glows when she shares her story.

Pathfinder David Lewine spent hours each day doing yoga for many years. Now, at age 86, and suffering from bladder cancer caused by contaminated water he ingested while serving in the Marines, he augments his yoga with daily exercise and lifting weights.

"Exercise likely works through several mechanisms," says Dr. Thomas Gill, director of the Yale Program on Aging. "Increasing physical activity will improve endurance; it benefits muscle strength and balance and reduces occurrence of serious fall injuries. It also provides a psychological benefit by lifting spirits."

Longevity research actually reveals a pleasant surprise: "A 2016 study found that elderly people who exercised for only 15 minutes each day, at an intensity level of a brisk walk, had a 22% lower risk of early death compared to people who did no exercise. A 2017 study found that exercising even just two days a week could lower risk for premature death. Researchers from McMaster University in Canada even found that breaking a sweat for just 60 seconds may be enough to improve health and fitness (as long as it's a tough workout)." [23]

In a study at the Mayo clinic, after 12 weeks, all the volunteers experienced improvements in fitness and could regulate their blood sugar. Those who weight-trained improved muscle mass and strength, while those who only did interval training improved endurance. The most surprising results came from the biopsied muscle cells: The youngest volunteers who exercised registered 280 regenerated genes while the oldest participants regenerated 400 genes!

As the saying goes, "if you don't use it, you lose it."

---

[23] Kluger, Jeffrey and Sifferlin, Alexandra, "How To Live Longer, Better*" TIME magazine, 2/15/18, p. 49

Exercise Keeps Aging Muscles and Immune Systems Young

A March 2018 article in *The New York Times* considered "How Exercise Can Keep Aging Muscles and Immune Systems Young" according to two studies, which tracked older, long-term cyclists who ride for fun.

Surprisingly, only 10 percent of people in the Western world over 65 actually work out regularly. An earlier study found that a group of men and women, 55 to 79, who had cycled for decades and continued to do so, compared considerably better physically and cognitively to a much younger group; in fact, the older group resembled those of 30-year-olds.

The two new studies mentioned, published in the journal, Aging Cell, looked closely at muscles and infection-fighting T cells, a major component of our immune system.

Both concluded that the older cyclists were healthier and biologically younger. The riders who tallied the most mileage had the healthiest muscles, no matter the age.

The aging cyclists had nearly as many new T cells as the young people, indicating the strong ability to prevent autoimmune reactions. All this said, it remained unclear whether picking up cycling at, let's say, 60, rather than at 40 or so, would have the same benefits. Nonetheless, clearly working our muscles retains strength and may improve our immunity.

Just Walk

Pathfinder Sarnie Ogus, 93, walks every day. Living in New York City, she loves to tread along the streets of Manhattan and the paths of Central Park while she connects with her body and her breathing. She also likes to connect with others—both human and canine—who walk the big city. "I'm amazed at how open people are," she says. "I guess we all need to connect." She loves to watch people and their dogs, and to simply stand in awe at the great diversity.

When I lived in New York City, I literally walked everywhere! When I moved with my family to the country, I stopped walking and fell into the all too common but unhealthy practice of driving everywhere. Now, to stay fit I have to "plan" my walks in the woods or along the Hudson River.

There are city dwellers who choose to remain in a metropolitan area well into old age, simply because the fast pace and energy of city life keeps them stimulated and vital. In fact, currently, 80% of Americans ages 65 and older are now living in metropolitan areas. According to the World Health Organization, by 2030 an estimated 60% of all people over age 60 will live in cities. While older urbanites might lose a little sidewalk speed and have to work harder to get up and down subway stairs, cities increasingly rank high on both doctors' and seniors' lists of the best places to age gracefully.

Even if we enjoy the city, many of us long for nature to give ourselves a taste of tranquility, to open our senses and our hearts to the awe-inspiring beauty of the natural world, of which we are an integral part. In his book Aging as Spiritual Practice, Zen Buddhist priest Lewis Richmond shares that he takes walks as a spiritual exercise in gratitude for the air, the trees, the birds, even the falling leaf or the single rock at his feet.

He suggests taking a notebook and a writing implement along when walking in the woods, up a mountainside, or on a beach, and jotting down such moments of gratitude. Taking notes can refresh our memories of the things we notice, witness, and observe while in a grateful state of mind. Perhaps such notes to self might even serve as the basis for a meditation.

Being Moved

This brings me to the importance of *being* moved, allowing our emotions to rise and fall, for instance, while engaging in a deep conversation, lingering before a particularly beautiful or provocative work of art, witnessing an absorbing film, play, or dance performance, or listening to a piece of music that may touch our hearts or make us feel like jumping out of our seat to "boogie on down"!

As Atul Gawande, the Indian American surgeon, writer, and public health researcher, reminds us in his book *Being Mortal*, the quality of our older years depends heavily on attitude and purpose. When we're engaged in life and appreciate being alive, he says, we live with grace. This doesn't mean practicing a false idealism. Rather, Dr. Gawande encourages us to do what we can to accept the aging process, to focus less on our ailments and more on what brings us joy. A bit of complaining or kvetching along the way, especially among peers, need not be a pity party but an opportunity to release our anxieties and disappointments without blaming others and, especially, without blaming ourselves. Shame and blame serve no purpose; it is purpose and gratitude that will create a life worth living until the end.

Cultivating the Seeds of the Sixth Grace: Moving and Being Moved

Studies show that just five minutes each hour, if we get up and walk a few steps, our health improves. When you go on errands, consider walking the aisles in the supermarket, look for a while before you choose what to buy. Park your car a distance from the mall entrance instead of trying for that spot close to it.

1. **Choose exercise that you enjoy:** With such an array of choices—yoga, walking, hiking, dancing, weightlifting, swimming, cycling—do

whatever feels right in your body and invites you to exercise and be joyful.

2. **Try Tai Chi:** My teacher, the Tai Chi master, Chungliang Al Huang, begins each course with a stance that joins heaven and earth through the body. Try it: Stand with legs apart with both arms extended upward toward the sky and your eyes looking up as well. Greet the day or just a few minutes with this stance and imagine the energy of the universe being pulled down through your fingers into your body and going through your feet, planting you into the earth. Breathe and smile. Note: One of the most-watched TED talks features social psychologist Amy Cuddy, who teaches this stance. She claims that it saved her life, renewing her confidence and personal power.

3. **Be consistent:** Make your chosen exercise a dedicated practice.

4. **Spend time in nature, without an agenda:** Notice your surroundings, practice mindfulness, open your senses and your heart—be moved!

5. **Find a group to share movement activities with:** Walk together, share a yoga class or any form of exercise, such as bicycling or dancing. It's often easier to stay motivated if you're part of a group.

Online Resources for Moving and Being Moved

Inspirational Stories:

https://www.facebook.com/nasdaily/videos/1095795007239317/

Travel:

Road Scholars (Formerly Elder Hostels): https://www.roadscholar.org

Living with other seniors when you travel abroad:

https://seniorplanet.org/the-freebird-club-a-new-airbnb-just-for-seniors/

Solo Travel: https://solotravelerworld.com

Spirituality:

The Elder Spirituality Project - http://www.spiritualityandpractice.com/projects/elder-spirituality/overview

SEVENTH GRACE

Nurturing the Body, the Temple of the Divine

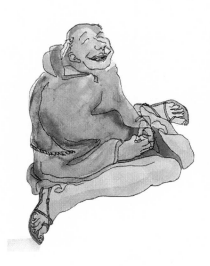

"Be aware when things are out of balance."
—Lao Tzu, *Tao Te Ching*

"There is only one temple in the world and that is the human body. Nothing is more sacred then that noble form."
—Novalis (Fredrich von Leopold)

"To lengthen thy life, lessen thy meals."
—Ben Franklin

"Love is love, not to be defined or described by the mind as exclusive or inclusive. Love is its own eternity: it is the real, the supreme, the immeasurable."
—Jiddu Krishnamurti, *The First and Last Freedom*

"He who will have no time for health today may have no health for time tomorrow."
—Anonymous

"Eat food. Not too much. Mostly plants."
—Michael Pollan

"Our food should be our medicine and our medicine shall be our food."
—Hippocrates

"The secret of staying young is to live honestly, eat slowly, and lie about your age."
—Lucille Ball

"Aging doesn't bother me; it never did. You just breathe in and breathe out."
—Pathfinder Iris Alster

We've learned a lot about consciously aging from our first six Graces, including managing and reducing stress through nurturing relationships, the benefits of mindfulness and pursuing a passion, living simply with gratitude and humor, and the importance of avoiding a sedentary lifestyle. In the Seventh Grace, we focus on nourishment and care of the body.

The human body is a miraculous machine. Some say it's the temple to the Divine, given to us to care for; others consider it a living mechanism. No matter how we choose to conceive of our physical form it must be properly maintained, and the responsibility is ours. How do we best ensure our body's capacity to sustain life and shelter our spirit for many years to come?

The last of our Seven Graces focuses on the three essential sources that support the body's vital energy: nourishing food and drink; plenty of fresh, clean water and air; and relationships that nourish our soul.

For most of us, by the time we reach our elder years, our bodies have begun to show the strain of living. The time has come to maintain the temple, our essential home on earth, or to allow our spirit to naturally depart and find a new home. (It's the law of physics! Energy can't be created or destroyed, only converted to another form.)

EMELINA EDWARDS
AGE 79

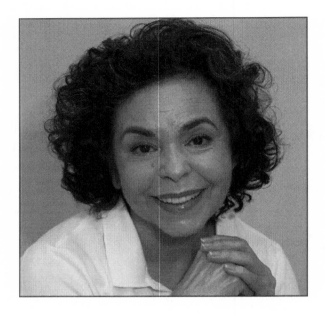

*Some people actually enjoy lifting weights, like fitness coach, **Emelina Edwards** of New Orleans, who at 79 years old, at the time of this writing, is still happily lifting over 100 pounds over her head while squatting. Along with weightlifting, Emelina also keeps fit and happy by eating whole foods, no meat, and a mostly plant–based diet, except for the ubiquitous, fresh seafood of her home city. She cherishes her meditation routine and says that she considers her clients, those with whom she's counseled and coached for over 20 years, her family, along with her sons, their wives, and her grandchildren. Emelina works out in her own home*

studio every single day, even when she may not feel like doing it, because she loves the results.

How did Emelina find her path? When she was in her fifties, her husband abandoned her and their children, leaving her destitute without marketable skills. Emelina fell into a deep depression. In her state of helplessness she realized that the only control she had was control over her body and her health. She was determined to become strong and healthy by getting her body in shape. She knew instinctively that this would re-shape her life. This reinvention of herself led her ultimately to become a fitness coach and nutritional advisor, an author, and a motivational speaker.

As a health coach, Emelina instructs her clients in diet, nutrition, exercise, weight, and meditation to help them age gracefully. Emelina shares her practical wisdom and life lessons in her two books: Forever Fit and Fabulous—A Guide to Health and Vigor at 70 and Beyond *and* The Journey to Self Esteem.

Many of my clients claim that their understanding of the natural cycles inherent in Chinese medicine have made it easier to observe their own body and its natural rhythm as well as to become more conscious of how to nourish theselves in accordance with the seasonal cycles. They believe that understanding these connections to nature has helped them pay closer attention to eating right, exercising regularly, and seeking emotional nourishment.

The Ancient Chinese Model of Health

Traditional Chinese medicine offers a system for living that encapsulates both thinking and being and states its principles lyrically and with profound pragmatism. The unfolding metaphor of Wholeness, intrinsic to Chinese medicine and represented by the yin/yang symbol, challenges us to seek and accept our ever-changing journey through life. For me, this ancient and venerable approach to health and healing has provided a roadmap to consciousness that I could share with others.

When I was young, my seeking nature led me to explore healing traditions around the world and introduced me to my life's work as an acupuncturist and practitioner of Chinese medicine. I learned a great deal by immersing myself in the ancient wisdom of the *Neijing, The Yellow Emperor's Classic of Medicine*, one of the most important Taoist texts and the supreme authority on the practice of traditional Chinese medicine. Attributed to the great Huang Di, the Yellow Emperor, who reigned during the third millennium BCE, the *Neijing* is believed to be nearly 4,000 years old. And yet, it offers timeless wisdom.

One of my favorite passages appears on the very first page, when Huang Di asks his minister and guide, Qi Bo, why people in the days of old enjoyed longer, happier lives. Does the world change from one generation to the next, he asks, or have people forgotten how to live in harmony with the enduring laws of nature? Qi Bo gently answers the young emperor's questions, speaking at length about the dramatic changes in lifestyle and philosophy that have contributed to the predicament of chronic disease, premature aging, and a general state of disharmony— all of which linger to this very day.

"In the past," Qi Bo observes, "people practiced the Tao, the Way of Life." They understood the principle of balance, of yin and yang, as represented by the transformation of the universal energies. Thus, they formulated practices such as Dao-In (an exercise that combines stretching, massaging, and breathing to promote energy flow) and meditation to help maintain and harmonize themselves with the universe. They ate a balanced diet at regular times, arose and retired at regular hours, avoided overstressing their bodies and minds, and refrained from overindulgence of all kinds. They maintained well-being of body and mind; thus, it is not surprising that they lived over 100 years.

These days, people have changed their way of life. They drink wine as though it were water, indulge excessively in destructive activities, drain their jing—the body's essence that is stored in the kidneys—and deplete their chi (vital energy). They do not know the secret of conserving their energy and vitality. Seeking emotional excitement and momentary pleasures, people disregard the natural rhythm and order of the universe. They fail to regulate their lifestyle and diet as well as sleep improperly. So, it is not surprising that they look old at 50 and die soon after.

To better focus on the Seventh Grace as a guide to nurturing your body and soul, your temple of the divine, I'm pleased to share with you the basic principles of Chinese medicine. It's my hope that you, too, may come to appreciate, if you haven't already, your body's own innate wisdom, so that you can better maintain it as you grow older.

The Buddhist sages speak of emptiness as openness, which allows us to receive. When we are in right relation, we give and receive reciprocally. With this in mind, I ask you to empty yourself, even temporarily, of preconceived beliefs, and consider what may be, for you, a new model for well-being so that you can, if you choose to, receive its time-honored wisdom.

A favorite teaching story illustrates this thought:

A university professor approached a master hoping to learn the nature of Zen. "I know a great deal about the workings of the physical world," the scholar explained, "but perhaps you could add to my knowledge by offering some thoughts about the nature of the spiritual world."

"Let us have a cup of tea," said the master, "and then we shall talk." The professor held out his cup as the master poured, filling the cup to the brim and then continuing to pour while the tea spilled onto the floor.

"It is overflowing!" protested the professor. "No more will go in!"

"Yes, it is so," said the master. "Just as this cup is full to overflowing, so is your mind filled with opinions and speculations, leaving no room to receive the teachings. Only when you empty your cup, can we begin."

The Basics of Chinese Medicine - a very simplified introduction

The Tao (Go with the flow!)

Taoist philosophy forms the philosophical heart of traditional Chinese medicine. It's described in the *I Ching* (Book of Changes) and the *Tao Te Ching* by Lao Tzu, as an invisible web of interconnections that support life, infusing all of nature with balance and harmony. In the *Tao Te Ching*, Lao Tzu states:

There was something formless and perfect before the universe was born. It is serene. Empty. Solitary. Unchanging. Infinite. Eternally present. It is the mother of the universe. For lack of a better name, I call it the

Tao. It flows through all things, inside and outside, and returns to the origin of all things.

Yin and Yang (Finding and keeping your balance)

While the Tao expresses unity—oneness, the source, the essential nature of the universe—two primordial powers, *yin* and *yang*, emerge out of this unity and alternate in the perpetual process, or cycle, of change between increase and decrease, expansion and contraction, fullness and emptiness. Yin and yang are not absolute opposites; they are simply two halves of a whole. Taoist philosophy teaches that everything in life, both literally and figuratively, contains its opposite. Over time, each half is continually transformed into the other in a continual cycle of change.

Throughout Chinese thought and medicine, when the complementary powers of yin and yang flow and interact in harmony, balance emerges. When the yin and yang dynamic is unequal, that is, out of balance, conflict ensues. The Chinese imagine the yin and yang as ever-changing aspects of a unified whole. This suggests that life lived within a changing universe requires a perpetual rebalancing from within, to align with the ineffable Tao, or the "All That Is."

The Western mindset all too often takes an "either/or" view of reality and dismisses the eternal, vital, flowing dynamic of the yin and yang. Such an approach perpetuates a hierarchical principle that wields power over people, creatures, and natural resources. The Tao lauds both the creative energy of the yang and the equally essential yielding, receptive way of the yin, which offers the greatest source of wisdom for human beings.

Chi (Tapping into the life-force)

The nature of *chi*, or energy, embodies the yin-yang dynamic. Yin carries the negatively charged molecule; yang carries the positively charged molecule. The two interact to produce electricity, or chi, the vibrational energy in Chinese medicine. Chi manifests the life force in nature and energizes all living creatures. As long as the energy flows, health and well-being thrive. When the chi is obstructed or blocked, dis-ease follows.

Chi does not take concrete physical form. It emanates a force field as when we "feel" another person's energy, or even that of a place. The Chinese consider the Earth a living organism with a unique force field, permeated with energy channels that perpetually change and move through its surface.

In traditional Chinese medicine, the human body, like the Earth, has underground channels, similar to blood vessels and nerves but invisible to the naked eye. These pathways carry chi, or energy, through the body, and their currents have the capacity to nourish all the human organs as well as the emotions. The points along these channels that vibrate close to the body's surface are the acupoints, which, with the application of delicate needles or pressure, provide access to a body's energy and can affect the flow of that energy through a particular channel, affecting its related organ.

When we begin to understand chi as the reservoir of energy that it can be—a regenerative, but too-often depleted resource—we learn to accept life as unpredictable and ever changing. To thrive and remain balanced we must learn to adapt to this principle. From the perspective of traditional Chinese medicine, nourishing the health of our body nourishes the health of the planet. When we're "in sync" with what makes us feel alive, we align with our natural flow and contribute to the Earth's well-being.

Building Blocks of our Vital Energy

Traditional Chinese medicine teaches three essential forms of energy, which combine to create the energies which support our physiological functioning (Ching chi) as well as our immune system (Wei chi):

1. the energy we receive from air;
2. the energy we receive from food and drink, particularly water; and
3. the energy we receive from nurturing relationships.

In essence, we can nurture our bodies with "right air," "right food," and "right relation."

Da chi (Wake up and smell the roses!)

"Breathing in, I calm my body and mind. Breathing out, I smile."

—Thich Nhat Hanh

The energy we receive from air is called Da chi. We acquire Da chi from the air we breathe, as the lungs circulate it throughout the body. We nurture it by breathing fresh air and can further support it by practicing very gentle breathing exercises.

In 1982, the Japanese government introduced "forest bathing" (an excellent example of applying Da chi in daily life), as an effective therapy. It was based on the idea that when in nature we thrive and when removed from nature our bodies weaken, age, and even become sick. From 2004 to 2012, Japan invested millions of dollars to research "forest bathing" by studying how hundreds of people in a variety of contexts and in different forests across the country responded to their forest walks. Though their studies were not limited to elders, physician Qing Li and his colleagues at Nippon Medical School found that walking through forests enhances an individual's outlook while also increasing longevity, improving quality of life, and also productivity at work. Clearly, forest bathing incorporates moving (walking) and the breathing of fresh air that has been processed by the plants and trees, to remove toxins and CO_2 for transformation into healthy, oxygen-rich air.

In urban centers across the globe, city planners carefully bring nature to the city to create enclaves of comforting, supportive, even inspiring environments. What would walking in Paris be without her abundant public gardens in which to relax? Or, New York City without the sanctuary of Central Park or the High Line?

We take in the life-force through our breath. In fact, the very word for breathing in is *in-spiration*, literally the taking in of spirit. Nearly all of our Pathfinders speak of their need for clean air, taking walks in nature, and focusing on their breath for centering and meditation. My teacher Chungliang Al Huang exemplifies the benefits to be derived from using our lungs (and our noses, mouths, and limbs) to tap into the life force. Huang lives the Tao. Throughout his life he has embraced his own connection to the life force through breath and movement and has helped thousands of others do the same.

Gu chi (Feeding the body, feeding the soul)

"The Chinese don't make any distinction between food and medicine."

—Lin Yutang

The energy we receive from food and drink is called Gu chi. We support it with a healthy diet. (In other words, "You are what you eat.") The digestive organs—the stomach, spleen, and pancreas—distribute *Gu chi* throughout the body. The Chinese consider eating fresh food, in season, to be essential to good health as well as moderation of quantity, and always plenty of water. The body must break down the food we consume in order to absorb its nutrients and the vital energy locked within, and to effectively discard its waste. This vital energy, then, must be distributed throughout the body.

Our Pathfinders speak of healthy eating as essential to their longevity.

Shen chi (Getting and giving the love we need)

"Any time that is not spent on love is wasted."

—Tasso

The energy we receive from nurturing relationships is called Shen chi. We obtain Shen chi from our personal connections with family, friends, and the natural world. The heart distributes it throughout the body. Nourishing relationships feed *shen chi*; toxic ones deplete it.

Pathfinder David Lewine, malnourished both emotionally and spiritually from his past, was able to transcend his traumatic past and restore his well-being when he discovered meditation and kindred friendships. Now, David gives back by volunteering to help those in need.

Note: Refer to the Second Grace, "Finding Your Tribe," for a practical discussion of the great benefits of cultivating nourishing relationships.

Entering the Blue Zones

Blue Zones are regions of the world renowned for having many more individuals living well past 100 then other cultures. These cultures share an abundance of fresh air, fresh food in season, and notably close social networks.

Ecuador

In 1981, the physician and medical journalist Morton Walker, DPM, conducted a series of studies on the health of the Vilcabamba people in Ecuador and wrote effusively of what he found: "In the Western Hemisphere, a place exists where degenerative diseases seldom if ever affect the population. The people have no heart disease, no cancer, no diabetes, no stroke, no cirrhosis, no senility, no arteriosclerosis, nor any other morbid conditions connected with an interruption in blood flow that are commonly responsible for illness, disability, and death among industrialized people. Since they don't die of degenerative diseases, the inhabitants of this place are able to live the full complement of mankind's years—more than a century. Vilcabamba is a veritable paradise on earth...Over the years the Sacred Valley has been variously called 'The Land of Eternal Youth,' 'The Valley of Peace and Tranquility,' and 'The Lost Paradise.' It has been given these labels because of the valley's solitude, serenity, clean air, dazzling sun, nearly constant blue sky, pure mineral drinking water, helpful neighbors, lack of illness, and a kind of ubiquitous beauty that penetrates to one's soul and provides a sense of well-being."[24]

Japan

Elder Okinawans in Japan attribute their healthy, long lives to nutritious, wholesome foods. They cite familiar proverbs such as "Food should nourish life—this is the best medicine." and "One who eats whole food will be strong and healthy."

According to researchers of the Okinawa Centenarian Study, their elders' diet consists of:

- Low calories
- Good carbohydrates from whole grains, vegetables, and fruits
- Nothing processed
- Seasonal fresh foods, locally grown
- Low amounts of naturally sourced fat
- Protein derived from beans, peas, whole grains, seeds, and nuts

These findings mirror the diets of the world's healthiest people who live the longest. Okinawans follow common sense and rarely overeat, preferring to

---

[24] Morton Walker, *Secrets of Long Life* (Devin-Adair, 1984), cited in *Vilcabamba: The Sacred Valley of the Centenarians* (CIS Publishing, 2004), pp. 31– 32.

stop at 80% full, which accommodates the fact that it takes about 20 minutes for stretch-receptors in the stomach to communicate to the brain how "full" we are.

In fact, a 1997 study cited in *The New England Journal of Medicine* points to the Okinawans' low-calorie intake as relating directly to their health and longevity. Overall, many researchers have clarified the relationship between low-caloric, high-nutrient diets as a major factor in healthy long life. Dr. Roy Walford, a top gerontologist at UCLA who conducted conclusive research funded by the National Institutes of Health across three decades, wrote:

"We can with an order of probability bordering on certainty extend maximum human life span by means of a calorically restricted optimal nutrition diet. There is now abundant hard (well-controlled and experimental) evidence…that a low-calorie diet that provides optimum nutrition will greatly extend average and maximum life spans, postpone the onset and decrease the frequencies of most or all of the "diseases of aging," maintain biomarkers at levels younger than chronological age, maintain sexual potency, general vitality, ability to engage in sports into advanced age, and delay deterioration of the brain." [25]

---

[25] Roy Walford, M.D., *Beyond the 120–Year Diet: How to Double Your Vital Years* (Four Walls Eight Windows: New York, 2000), p. 89.

Pakistan

The food varieties that the Hunzan people grow on the fertile terraces in Pakistan have been called another great wonder of the world. The Hunzans eat entirely from the land, what's natural, cyclically varying their food as it matures, varying diet with each season, with, of course, no pesticides. In addition to their famously nutritious and delicious apricots, they grow peaches, pears, apples, plums, grapes, cherries, mulberries, figs, and many types of melons. They also harvest wild berries and huge apples.

Hunzans eat substantial portions of vegetables, primarily greens, including mustard greens, spinach and lettuce; also root vegetables and a wide assortment of legumes, along with various squashes, including pumpkins. They also cultivate many culinary and medicinal herbs and grow flaxseeds, a staple of their diet.

As mentioned previously, the Hunzans choose to eat most of their food raw, which minimizes the need for cooking fuel and protects the foods' nutrients. The traditional Hunzan diet is very similar to those of the Okinawans, Abkhasians, and Vilcabambans. All four cultures consume very little meat and significant portions of whole grains. Their diets are very low in calories by Western standards. Protein and fat are primarily plant and vegetable derivatives, and all food is wholesome and locally grown. The older people in all four cultures exhibit very low rates of disease, and many have strong eyes and teeth. Add to all this a beautiful environment with clean air, water, and soil, and a thriving, supportive community—and you have four groups of elders who are well-nourished, both physically and emotionally.

In his 2012 book, *The Blue Zones*, Dan Buettner names four additional Blue Zones: Sardinia, Italy; Nicoya, Costa Rica; Loma Linda, California, and Ikaria, Greece—all of which herald clean air, nutritious food, and strong community.

Inflammation: How It Works and How to Avoid It

In Chinese medicine, when we interfere with our nourishment through poor diet, difficult relationships, and polluted air, stagnation ensues. This leads to inflammation.

Many scientists and health professionals assert that inflammation causes many diseases and promotes premature aging. It's important to note, however, that inflammation serves a natural purpose. Inflammation is the immune system's natural, healthy response to a foreign substance, such as a cold or flu virus or an infected wound. The body's inflammatory response often saves our lives, and helps the body overcome its challenge. The danger lies with chronic inflammation—such as that caused by habitual stress—when the adrenal glands over-release cortisol, an inflammatory stress hormone.

Sustaining good health depends on mindful awareness of the body's stress responses, both from diet and lifestyle, and choosing to reduce all forms of unnecessary stress. Without such attention across a long life, the dangers of chronic, prolonged inflammation increase.

The Gut and Inflammation

Maintaining a healthy intestinal tract, better known as "the gut," is a fundamental antidote to chronic inflammation, which creates oxidation, causing cells to age prematurely. The very latest studies reveal that, in addition to chronic stress, inflammation most often originates in the gut through what's called dysbiosis, an imbalance of microorganisms in the gastrointestinal tract.

Cells oxidize and age when they're inflamed; healthy foods support the production of good bacteria in the gut. Some examples include cruciferous vegetables like broccoli, kale, cabbage, and cauliflower; bananas, blueberries, beans, polenta, artichokes, and fermented plant-based foods. On the other hand, foods containing sugar, refined carbohydrates, and preservatives feed the inflammatory response within the human biome.

If we remove foods from our diet that promote inflammation we can calm and balance the bacteria, decrease the inflammation, and re-establish a healthy, probiotic internal environment. A happy gut promotes lucid brain function, boosts the immune system, and retards aging. In short, if you can't pronounce it, don't eat it.

Food Sensitivity and Inflammation

Eating a variety of foods is also vital to a healthy gut. Nature matures different foods at different times of year, so it's natural to rotate them in our diets. The immune system, however, is built to be wary of foreign proteins, which enter our body through the mouth. In fact, most pathogens enter the body through our food.

Seventy-five percent of our immune system centers in and around the gut because we must debilitate potentially harmful proteins. Fortunately, that's how the body works, but it remains up to us to practice due diligence and not exacerbate inflammation by eating foreign proteins, such as wheat and dairy, at every meal.

Also, our immune system is programmed to distinguish between self and other, allowing for seasonal variations in our diet. If we don't diversify our diet, the immune system learns to attack harmless protein, leading to chronic inflammation, which, in turn, can promote hyper-allergic reactions or even autoimmune disease. Such inflammation also accelerates aging.

Moderation Is Still Key

"In eating, a third of the stomach should be filled with food, a third filled with drink and the rest left empty."

—The Talmud

"A glutton digs his grave with his teeth."

—French Proverb

Letting go of dieting, especially if you're at a healthy weight, is more than reasonable. A 2016 study found that women over age 50 who started at a normal weight, but whose weight fluctuated due to dieting, earned no health benefit, including no less cardiac arrest.

Also in 2017, a study led by Dr. Frank Hu, chair of the Department of Nutrition at Harvard University's T.H. Chan School of Public Health, and published in *The New England Journal of Medicine*, declared that improving your diet just a little bit can help you live longer. The study found that the largest increase in healthy eating lowered the risk of death by 8-17%. The researchers concluded that swapping one serving of red or processed meat for nuts or legumes, such as beans, lentils, peas, and peanuts could create such a result.

All of the Pathfinders found diet to be essential to their longevity, differing only based on beliefs and body types. Their dietary considerations all included: cutting out or reducing sugar, eating less, not buying food with chemicals in them, and drinking plenty of water.

Staying Sexy at Any Age

For most elders, minor indulgences in food and drink are harmless and pleasurable, including sex! Remaining sexually active definitely increases basic life satisfaction, and, in some cases, also increases longevity.

Dr. Ruth Westheimer, age 92, is a long time, widely respected sex therapist, media personality, and author. 'Dr. Ruth' has taught at Princeton and Yale and has written over 40 books on sex and sexuality. She continues to strongly promote the physical and emotional health advantages of an active sex life well into the later years.

The research supports her. Studies show that human sexuality remains a driving force in elders, though it is often misunderstood. In fact, human beings are never too old to enjoy a healthy and happy sex life. Hormonal levels do, however, drop considerably after 60 and therefore libido dissipates, first, most noticeably in women. This appears to be more of a concern for older men who identify more readily with sexual performance while women (and some more aware men) adjust to sexuality later in life as an expression of affection, devotion, even a loving renewal of romance—a natural, regenerative part of life, where joy can be expressed and experienced. All this said, with the increase in elderhood of potential boredom, anxiety or fear, fatigue, and especially grief, an interest in sex can be repressed or forgotten.

Elder sex can actually have health benefits. For example, a study published in 2019 compared cognition to those between 50 and 89 who were or were not sexually active. Researchers determined that there is an association between sex and improved recall. Men showed more aptitude in remembering number sequences, while women had a better overall memory. [26]

But we don't only need studies to tell us whether older couples are enjoying each other sexually. The skin glows; the smile is genuine; there may even be a wry, knowing humor about it all. Even though sex for long-together couples changes when hormonal levels fall, the change can foster intimacy. Arousal need not occur only from heightened libido, visual stimulation, or fantasies. Arousal can emerge from being truly seen and known just as one is. Of course, there's a fine line, particularly for men. It's hard (no pun intended) for a man to have an erection if he's feeling vulnerable. But when such tenderness can be witnessed by a loving partner, arousal comes naturally (again no pun intended).

This reminds me of the story of an elderly former bathing beauty named Matilda who had just turned 90. When she was a girl, she'd won first place in a slew of pageants. Her talent had been swimming, so wearing a bathing suit had come very naturally.

---

[26] Hayley Wright, Rebecca A. Jenks, *Age and Ageing*, "Sex on the brain! Associations between sexual activity and cognitive function in older age," Volume 45, Issue 2, March 2016, pp. 313–317.

On the usual day her daughter Alice came to visit, Matilda asked her to help her pack.

"Wherever are you going, Mother?" her daughter asked, both bemused and a bit concerned.

"Ralph and I have decided to get married," Matilda announced. Not waiting for her daughter, who appeared frozen in place, to respond, she continued, "We're going on a honeymoon cruise to the Bahamas and I'll need lots of bathing suits," Matilda said, matter of factly, pointing to the dresser drawer near the rocker where Alice sat staring at her.

"Go ahead dear, please, open that bottom drawer for me."

Alice stood automatically, before kneeling to better open the low drawer. When she pulled it out, her audible gasp made her mother jump in her seat.

"Goodness, dear, didn't you know I'd saved my lucky suits?"

"Mother, there's nothing in this drawer but swimsuits."

"I know. I know. I love them all, but only choose the one-pieces. I've gotten too scrawny to hold up the bandeau without falsies. Good thing Ralph likes me just the way I am."

"That's most important, Mother."

"Thank you, dear, thank you for understanding."

Of course, Matilda was not likely to be off on a Caribbean cruise, but she and Ralph did get married. She married a younger man. Ralph was only 88.

"We don't stop playing because we get old, we get old because we stop playing."

—George Bernard Shaw

Cultivating the Seeds of the Seventh Grace: Nurturing Your Body, Your Temple of the Divine

To support diet and nutrition:

1. **Don't eat on the run.** Sit for your meal. Eat slowly and chew well to release all the digestive juices. Inflammation can occur when proteins seep into our body fluids due to incomplete digestion (leaky gut syndrome). When we eat slowly, mixing our food with saliva, the saliva and other enzymes break down the proteins. As the Zen proverb advises: "When you're eating, eat!"

2. **Eliminate most or all refined carbohydrates.** Restricting sugar and white flour is a good start.

3. **Avoid fried foods.** Use primarily extra virgin olive oil for cooking; bake, grill, roast, or sauté foods rather than frying.

4. **Avoid red meat.** It's difficult to digest and creates mucus in the system, which can slow down digestion and increase the burden on the

stomach and intestines. Substitute fish, chicken, or turkey (with skin removed) for red meat.

5. **Make animal protein a side dish, rather than an entrée.** Explore plant-based alternatives such as beans, chickpeas, lentils, and quinoa.

6. **Check all ingredients.** If you can't pronounce it, don't eat it. Artificial colors and most preservatives increase inflammation and the body stores them as fat.

7. **Buy organic, if possible.** Organic fruits and veggies may be more expensive, but the health benefits offset the extra cost.

8. **Increase your intake of raw, whole foods.** For example: raw, unsalted nuts and seeds; blueberries; oranges; bananas; avocados; carrots; cabbage; leafy greens such as kale, spinach, red leaf lettuce; bean sprouts; raw sauerkraut or yogurt.

9. **Eat whole grains.** These include amaranth, barley, brown rice, buckwheat, bulgur, corn, kamut, millet, oats, quinoa, rye, sorghum, spelt, wheat berries, and wild rice.

10. **Rotate your foods.** Just as nature provides diversity through the seasons, it's good to vary your diet with foods that are in season and to avoid eating the same thing every day. Studies

and ancient Chinese wisdom show that when we eat the same meals again and again, we develop food allergies, and inflammation. A recent article about Britain's Queen Elizabeth, titled "The Nine Foods You'll Never See Her Eat," emphasizes the importance of the "foods-in-season" rule. Never, ever offer the Queen strawberries in January! At 92 she eats only organic foods, in season, and no GMOs. Thank you, Your Majesty!

11. **Learn to reconnect with your body's innate wisdom.** Listen to your symptoms, your aches and pains. Ask yourself what your body is trying to tell you?

12. **Eat mindfully.** When eating out or craving a certain food that might not be good for you, listen to your body and ask yourself, "What will truly nourish me? How will I feel after I eat this?"

13. **Drink clean, non-carbonated water.** Preferably six to ten 8-ounce glasses per day. This helps detox the liver and kidneys.

14. **Breathe clean fresh air.** Make a commitment to spend time outside, preferably in nature, each day and simply breathe in the fresh air.

Online Resources for Nurturing Your Body:

Feeding Your Body:

Refer to articles on nutrition at the U.S. Department of Agriculture (USDA) website: https://www.nutrition.gov/subject/life-stages/seniors

Choosing what organics to eat: https://organic.org/the-dirty-dozen/

https://nutritionfacts.org - Strictly non-commercial, science-based public service provided by Dr. Michael Greger, providing free updates on the latest in nutrition research via bite-sized videos.

EPILOGUE

Living Unto Death and
Facing Our Mortality

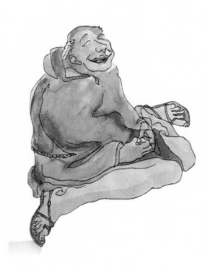

"As a well-spent day brings happy sleep, so life, well used, brings happy death."
—Leonardo da Vinci

"To be blessed in death one must learn to live. To be blessed in life, one must learn to die."
—Jesuit verse

Asilence, if not a sheer denial, inhibits our ability to face our mortality. Our pervasive technological world all too often eclipses the transcendent nature of death well recognized by ancient cultures. When we can accept our mortality not as a lapse in God's grace, but as a fact of nature (every living thing dies), we can more fully embrace our lives. Releasing our constrictive fears can transform our angst into awe, gratitude, and deep appreciation for all that we've lived and all that we are becoming. Levity about our mortality may even emerge. As Ram Dass once said, "Death is absolutely safe. Nobody ever fails at it."

> *"A monk, who is being chased by a tiger, comes to the edge of a cliff. As the tiger closes in on him, the monk notices a vine leading over the cliff and down into a precipice. Quickly, he crawls over the edge and lets himself down by the vine only to discover another tiger waiting for him below. Looking up, he observes a mouse gnawing away at the vine. Just then, he spots a luscious strawberry within arm's reach. The monk seizes the berry and eats it. Ah, how delicious it tastes!"*

As the story reminds us, our acceptance of death or, at the very least, our awareness of our own mortality, can open our hearts to awe and sheer gratitude for simply being alive.

Aging is a rite of passage. It takes courage, compassion, and community to live it well. We get stronger in the broken places or, as the poet Leonard Cohen wrote in his signature song, "Anthem," "There is a crack in everything....That's how the light gets in." Such awareness suggests that we are all in some way wounded. Perhaps if we could recognize our mutual wounds, our common humanity, we would awaken empathy and strengthen compassion around the world, fostering the healing of body, mind, and spirit for all.

This reminds me of a story in *Kitchen Table Wisdom*, a book by therapist and integrative medicine educator Rachel Naomi Ramen. The author recounts her experience with a 24-year-old high school and college athlete whose cancerous growth required surgical removal of his leg above the knee. One of the angriest patients Ramen had ever treated, overwrought with a sense of injustice and self-pity, this young man loathed everyone who was healthy. In their second therapy session, Ramen gave him a sketchbook and asked him to draw an image of his body. He drew an outline of what appeared to be a vase with a black, jagged crack running through it.

As time passed, the young man began to emerge from his isolation and self-pity by sharing his trauma with other wounded and despairing individuals. Through reaching out to others, he developed a sort of ministry. His own vulnerability heightened his empathy for the suffering of others. One day, he visited a young woman who had chosen to have both breasts removed to avoid a diagnosis that had taken many in her family. At first he couldn't reach her, but when he displayed his stump and danced around her room, he broke the ice. They laughed together, became fast friends, and eventually married.

On her final session with the young man, Ramen showed him his original drawing of the cracked vase. After studying it for some time, he remarked, "You know, it's really not finished." With a yellow crayon, he drew thick lines radiating out from the black crack. Pointing to the black line running through the vase, he explained that it was there—in the broken places—that the light shines through.

The "cracks" in his body, mind, and spirit did not diminish his strength but, instead, created the space and thus the potential for the light of compassion to shine through and illuminate his darkness. When he accepted himself, wounds and all, he renewed his soul.

Following are three individuals who served as my Pathfinders into death. Their lives and their passing transformed my own relationship with dying.

Vipassana: Glimpsing the Beyond

Back in the 1970s, I had a most humbling experience of death, where letting the light in meant surrendering to death. Having worked with healers and

193

healing modalities in the Philippines for some years, I had become known as a healer myself, though I wrestled with this title, aware of the danger of feeding my spiritual ego.

In anticipation of my return to the ashram in India, where I had previously stayed, a beloved friend shared that my reputation as a healer preceded me. People would be gathering in anticipation, hoping and praying that I could heal their fellow devotee, Vipassana, who had slipped into a coma from an inoperable brain tumor. (I learned that Vipassana means "insight into the true nature of reality.") Only 24, she and her twin brother, Viyogi, lived at the ashram.

Upon my arrival, I felt a bit anxious about the expectations awaiting me but walking on the familiar streets soothed me—the multicolored saris creating a sea of mutating color, titillating scents rising from sidewalk vendors, a myriad of incense, from sweet to strong. As the sun began to set, the air became quite chilly as we approached the ashram, gooseflesh emerging across my arms. A multitude of birds appeared, every size and color, flitting and flying about, when suddenly a hawk zeroed in on what I assumed was a rat, but instead came directly toward me, so close I had to swerve to avoid contact with it. A good omen...or bad?

Entering the ashram gates, pleading eyes looked through me as I approached, and my heart beat faster. As soon as possible, I arranged for Vipassana's friends and family, who anxiously awaited me, to meet in her room at the ashram that evening, where we would do a healing ceremony for her, though she lay inert in hospital.

Entering the room, many eyes latched upon mine, their gaze pleading, "Can you heal her?" "Will she be all right?" I introduced myself and hugged those whom I knew before explaining to the group of 40 people that our loving energy could support Vipassana's ability to heal herself. I shared that sending love and energy does not require the physical presence of those we are supporting, that Vipassana's energy permeated this space and we could connect to her from here.

I gestured for us to form a circle and join hands, and, for a few moments, to envision Vipassana—her voice, her laughter, her energy—and to allow her presence to penetrate each individual heart with the intention of our loving energy reaching into her.

To bring the vibrations to a higher octave, I invited the group to chant the sacred syllable "Om," with each exhale. Our voices rose in simultaneous harmony, intensifying the energy. When it had reached a crescendo, I asked the group to release their hands and to place them in front of them with palms up and to direct their love into Vipassana.

As I did the same, an intense, overwhelming pain filled my head, as if it would burst open. I had never felt such before and attempted to release the pain with my breath and again envision Vipassana, transmitting my thoughts of love and healing towards her. Again the intense pain in my head prevented me from communing with her.

As others completed their offering and slowly exited, exchanging hugs on the way out, I realized that I was drained. Thankfully her friends and family seemed content that they had contributed something toward Vipassana's healing, but I left with a deep sense of confusion and frustration.

Having been present at many healing sessions and led such sessions myself, I had not once felt such stabbing, unrelenting pain. What did it mean? I was determined to go to the hospital the next day to give Vipassana a hands-on healing.

After a morning of deep mediation and listening to my teacher's discourse, especially the silence between his words, I felt, on one hand, elated, but, leaving the ashram gates, trepidation washed over me.

Upon entering Vipassana's hospital room, her twin brother, Viyogi, greeted me with desperate eyes from across the room where he repeatedly pushed down on a manual respirator that provided his sister's breathing. I introduced myself and shared what had happened to me the evening before. Viyogi supported any offering I might make, grateful for whatever support I could provide.

I stood by Vipassana's side, the sounds of medical monitors beeping in the background and the hiss of air pumping into her lungs. I closed my eyes and entered my familiar healing trance, directing my full attention to Vipassana, sending love and energy through my hands. As I felt the force move through my body and into hers, the same excruciating head pain ensued. I attempted to fight it and found myself forcing the energy through. A voice came to me loud and clear, "Leave me alone, I'm not going back, it hurts too much!"

"You can do it; you can fight it," I responded silently. Again I heard what I believed to be Vipassana's voice, "No, leave me alone." (We seemed to meet in the silence, outside of her body.) I trusted her message and left the room, breaking down as I sat on the floor just outside her door, before soon realizing that I got such a headache because I was attempting to heal a vacant body. She had already passed over and merely hovered somewhere in the room. Who did I think I was to make such a demand on this dear soul? The experience left me shaken, and changed, for in all the years I'd cultivated my healing abilities, I'd never personally confronted this truth: it is not my will, but Thy will be done.

Upon deeper reflection back at the ashram, I realized, with the help of my teacher, that a door opens to the divine when a person is dying. When someone tries to keep the dying in his or her body, the "healer" or beloved cannot receive the gift from the dying one, a glimpse of the beyond.

Back at the hospital where the word had spread that no option remained, Viyogi deflated the respiration bag for the last time—no struggle, only gurgling, and a deep exhalation. An explosion of light suddenly filled the room. It seemed to permeate all of us, and we shared a deep sense of benediction. She had indeed passed into the light and gifted us with a momentary glimpse of the other side.

I learned through the pain of Vipassana's passing that we can do what can be done to promote healing, but we must remain humble. Healing has become, for me, a sacred path toward Oneness with All That Is, where the divine enters through the crack in the darkness, even unto death.

Embracing Mortality

My dear friend Deva Teerth, taught me about embracing mortality, one of the most important lessons of my life.

We met when we were in our early twenties, living in New York City's West Village, and both part of a meditation group. While meditating together, we became friends. Eventually, he shared with me his painful history with cancer of the upper palette. Surgery and chemo had successfully sent his cancer into remission. Though he had a plate in his upper palate, it was not noticeable and did not indicate that anything had been amiss. We enjoyed hiking, meditating, and socializing until I moved to India (where I lived for close to five years). Six months into my stay at the Ashram, Deva Teerth, too, became part of the community though he journeyed back and forth to the States. Our friendship remained strong.

In 1980, I moved back to the United States and settled in Woodstock, New York. Deva Teerth soon joined us in the Woodstock area, married his beloved, and we created a new community upstate.

A year later, Deva Teerth began experiencing pain in his jaw. He went back to the oncologist, who found that the cancer had returned and metastasized. He was told that this time there was not much that the Western medical community could do to help him. He continued to see oncologists and other physicians to explore possible treatment options, but always came up short. Nonetheless, Deva continued his meditation practice, consulted alternative healing practitioners, and all in all did what he could to support his immune response. Still, the cancer continued to grow.

Through a meditation group he learned of the work of Stephen and Ondrea Levine and the Center for Living Your Dying, which they had created in Santa Fe, New Mexico. It had become clear that short of a miracle, Deva Teerth would likely die within six months, and he very much wanted to consciously leave his body. So he moved into the Levines' center and sent us pictures and audiotapes of his process. Facing death amplified his each and every moment.

I remember the film he sent us shortly before he died. He sat on the side of the nearby river, making a fire, and placing in the flames all those relics from his past that he had once felt a strong attachment to. This ritual, he told me, reminded him of the transient nature of life itself. His face had been contorted from the cancer, but he was relatively pain-free due to both gentle medication and his meditation practice. After his ritual cleansing from the past, my friend looked deeply into the camera and spoke to the audience that would see the film after he had departed. His meditation on life-and-death implored all those watching to never forget to experience the exquisite Now.

"You need not have terminal cancer or be facing the imminent threat of death to experience that which is totally available to you in this very moment. I have no past or future. If there is but one gift I can share with you, it would be simply to enjoy every moment of your life because that's all there is! It can be filled with love as I am filled at this very moment."

Those were the last words that I heard from him. I knew that his life had been perfect as it was, even though dying in one's 40's is sad and untimely. I heard soon after that Elizabeth Kübler-Ross had been with him at his death, and that she had commented that she was jealous of his sublime letting go.

My friend's message of living fully until the end invited this epilogue.

Living *All* of Life

More recently, I lost another friend, Dr. John Stine, who also lived life to the fullest. When we met, about ten years ago, he was still a practicing psychiatrist, psychoanalyst, professor, and also a prominent jazz clarinetist. John loved music and had hoped when young to attend Julliard, but his future father-in-law convinced him that he couldn't support a family as a musician, so he went on to become a physician and through the war trained in psychiatry.

Shortly after befriending John, I learned of his pulmonary fibrosis diagnosis, a life-threatening disease of the lung. John was by far the most positive person I'd ever known. Approaching 80, he had to abandon his clarinet because he simply didn't have the breath any longer. So, what did he do? He took up guitar. And, when he became weaker still, he played his music on a keyboard. He also continued to attend concerts, to read, and to learn. John lived such an enriched life!

Whenever we got together we'd talk with great enthusiasm about everything on our minds and in our hearts. I had asked him to be one of my Pathfinders for this book, which he, of course, agreed to do, though often reminded me that he might not live to do it, all the while living fully.

I'd give him my pep talk about our mind's ability to reverse disease and he'd listen, not disputing my ideas, but saying always that he had no fear of death and intended to live a full life until he took his last breath. He did become a client near the end of his life when the pain from coughing had become excruciating. I do hope I helped ease his suffering a bit.

I learned a great deal from my friend John. From what his wife told me, he died peacefully, accepting death as the inevitable culmination of a life well lived. I spoke to friends of his at his funeral who told me that they had never met such a generous person.

One might retire, leave a job, but need never leave the sphere of learning. My ill but remarkably vital friend felt dismayed that rather than truly engaging life, he saw so many of the people he knew automatically attending cultural events but rarely truly participating in creative endeavors themselves. He believed, as I do, that learning is living, and living is learning. When we stop learning, we stifle growth and evolution, sabotaging our life force.

Assuaging Fear of Death: New Studies

In chapter three, the "Third Grace: Practicing Mindfulness," where we covered the great benefits of mindfulness, I mentioned author Michael Pollan's latest book, *How To Change Your Mind: The New Science of Psychedelics*, in which he explores the new research in psychedelic therapy. He notes the experiments that first piqued his interest, which occurred at Johns Hopkins, UCLA, and New York University, simultaneously in 2010, where terminal cancer patients volunteered to take a psychedelic drug for a single guided journey, this to assuage their fears of death. The results were overwhelmingly positive, with some individuals ranking the experience as "one of the most meaningful in their lives," and even one-third of those participating in the study describing the experience as the most meaningful of their entire life. Over a full year later, the positive results essentially held, marked by improved attitudes, heightened senses of well-being, and even changes in behavior.

An earlier study conducted in 2006 by the same Johns Hopkins team revealed that a high dose of psilocybin could create a mystical experience akin to a spiritual revelation. Such work echoes similar experiments begun but abandoned back in the 1950s and 1960s. Such positive new findings promise relief for many individuals suffering unnecessarily from the fear of death and other stultifying conditions.

More recently Pathfinder Janet Hariton, who trusts the space between worlds, said during our interview, "I believe that transitioning through death can be much less frightening than coming through the birth canal. When we throw off this mortal coil, we are free."

Filled with gratitude for the regenerative value of all Seven Graces, learning through my own early challenges of aging and enlightened by the generosity of my clients, my interviewees, my friends, and, of course, my family—my wife and my son—living is an art in itself; we master it less through our accomplishments and more through our feelings and our awareness. When we are present to our life, embracing it wholeheartedly even through hardship, we live meaningfully, consciously, even unto death.

That's what I've learned so far about "how to die young, as late in life as possible."

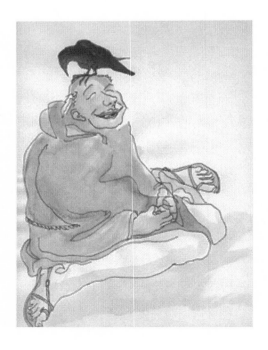

ENDNOTES

Elderhood in Western Culture: Yesterday & Today

During the Industrial Revolution, elders in Europe and North America lost their honored place in society as modern machines rendered them increasingly more and more useless. By 17th- and 18th-century Colonial times, the Puritans, who dominated most every aspect of social thinking, perpetuated the belief that people lived to old age because God chose them to lead. Not many among the colonists could read and those who could, usually the elders, earned great respect as the wise among them, looked to as mentors and teachers of traditional values.

Because they were the primary landowners with extended families in an agricultural society, the elders held the greatest wealth and therefore the greatest power. A patriarchal culture ruled the day where the fathers held power in government, over land, and over local farms. Though their positions demanded respect, the men in authority were often revered in fear and resentment. By the 19th century in America, industrialization in full swing, the sons of these land-owning patriarchs left rural gentlemen farms for the cities to gain necessary expertise for the ever-changing times.

Allegiance to traditional values waned as new generations surpassed the education of their elders and extended families broke away, ultimately evolving into more nuclear family constellations eager to live more progressive lives. Over time, the quest for technological advancement among the young left elders without significant roles.

What do we do with an older population rendered useless by an industrial society? We warehouse elders in isolated facilities, such as nursing homes, if the money runs out, and in assisted living and retirement communities, if there's a pension or savings or the kids' have funds to share. In any case, elders can all too often become victims of discrimination based on age. This dismissal of the elderly also condones a youth-centered society, where aging is looked down-upon. Such attitudes dissuade the young and even middle-aged from the reality of their own aging and death.

The "forever young," treadmill denies the bountiful freedom of old age, what the ancient Greek philosopher, Epicurus, considered the pinnacle of life. We are given the gift of youth, he said, but the passion and wisdom of age!

It's natural for older people to feel that more life is behind than ahead of them, but we too often "retire away" our elders rather than encouraging them to share their knowledge. It is exciting to see the emerging trend in our culture that's shifting the negative construct that has created a life sentence of retirement. We can now look at this valuable time with fresh eyes.

We might best ask when we approach our own retirement age, "What do I want to do with the rest of my life that will be meaningful?" "What can I give back?" "What does the world need from me?"

Aging is an opportunity. We can choose to embrace each day anew, embrace our pleasure, our creative passions, and learn "how to die young as late in life as possible," growing old gracefully, being who we truly are.

For better and worse, Western society has undergone another cultural shift in recent decades. Yet some of that norm-busting 1960s ethos remains. When it comes to our perceptions of aging, we are free to reject the idea that once you pass age 60, you will gradually withdraw from society, get sick and die. On the contrary, we can choose to stay as healthy as possible, for as long as possible—physically, emotionally, mentally, and spiritually—aging gracefully.

Egalitarianism Promotes Good Health & Longevity

Since 1980, disparity in incomes across the United States has increased the divide between rich and poor to the point that the nation's elite, the top one percent, now own more wealth than the bottom 90% combined. Until that time, U.S. social norms favored equality, strong labor unions, and progressive taxation. The nearly four decades that have sanctioned tax cuts for the rich, the decimation of regulation of industries that promote dangers to our climate, and the undercutting of government programs for the less fortunate have created a cultural divide that gravely impacts health, leaving some 44 million people without health insurance and another 35 million with inadequate coverage.

Medicare and Medicaid provide government-sponsored health care for the aged and infirm, however, how long will such entitlement programs survive in a country careening toward a trillion-dollar national debt?

Studies have shown that the larger the gap between rich and poor, the less healthy a nation will become.

An egalitarian society intends to satisfy its peoples' basic needs, promote community, trust, and mutual cooperation. People look out for each other. This well-lived philosophy decreases stress and encourages good health. Japan, for example, has the greatest life expectancy of any nation on earth—Okinawa with the greatest life expectancy in all of Japan. Though the Japanese smoke heavily, it is likely the equitability of its economic policies—the most fair and impartial of all the world's prosperous nations—that reveals the key to their peoples' longevity.

After World War II, General Douglas MacArthur exemplified an egalitarian approach in his supervision of Japan's reconstruction. He required the Japanese government to implement the following three essential things:

1. **demilitarization**, that is, to eliminate their army

2. **democratization**, including constitutionally providing for a representative democracy, free universal education, the right of labor unions to organize and to engage in collective bargaining, the right of women to vote, and the right of everyone to a decent life

3. **decentralization**, which intended to split up the family dynasties that had run the corporations controlling the country. MacArthur mandated a maximum wage for business and corporate leaders and implemented a land reform program considered the most successful in history. He essentially had the wealth redistributed, which leveled the playing field.

These measures initiated the most rapid increase in health and longevity ever documented in any major country in world history. Postwar Japan became a nation that cherished egalitarianism.

If only we, in America, cared less about winning or losing, about being number one, and more about each other and the simple yet awesome qualities of life itself. If only we, in America, could embrace the notion that health and well-being do not rely on financial riches or attractiveness but rather on redefining the meaning of aging, the meaning of family, the importance of a meaningful purpose or passion, living in the present, continuing to move the body, and always clean air, clean water, nourishing food, and nurturing relationships.

Diving Deeper into Mind over Matter & Placebos

In Joe Dispenza's book, *You Are the Placebo*, he shares that the term "placebo" was originally used in the portion of Psalm 116 that opens the Catholic vespers of the dead. Traditionally families hired "mourners" to exaggerate the lament in order to please the family of the deceased. And in the nineteenth century physicians began to give bogus pills to individuals with conditions that they couldn't cure, reportedly with often-good results.

The modern use of placebo began in 1955 with the publication in *The Journal of the American Medical Association* of an article by Dr. Henry K. Beecher called "The Powerful Placebo." The author recounted his experience as an Army surgeon during World War II. While tending to the wounds of the soldiers, he ran out of morphine. Knowing the pain and shock could kill them, he told his patients that he was injecting them to ease pain for surgery when, in fact, he used a saline solution. It astounded him that during surgery a good many of those patients appeared free from pain—a testament to the power of the mind to create reality.

After the war, Dr. Beecher repeated this process, noting that patients' conditions improved when they were encouraged to feel better. This led to clinical trials, which replicated and further documented the results of his wartime experiments.

The opposite situation, known as the "nocebo effect," occurs when subjects are told that a certain substance may harm them. (Nocebo means "I will harm.") When they believe this potential outcome, it has been shown to actually manifest. For example, take the case of a graduate student who became depressed upon breaking up with his girlfriend. He enrolled in an experimental clinical trial for a new anti-depressant drug. He had experienced side effects a number of years earlier and enrolled in the study to secure a new medication. When another trauma occurred, he was rushed to the ER. He exhibited all the symptoms of poisoning—rapid pulse, depressed blood pressure, pallor, and vomiting. To the doctors' surprise, his bloodwork came back normal. He had been taking the placebo, a sugar pill, which had become a nocebo because of his firm belief. The young man's symptoms abated as soon as this was explained to him.

It has long been the case that when studying experimental drugs or formulas to prove their worthiness as potential treatments, researchers must account for the placebo effect, as it is often responsible for 30-33% of the study's outcome; that is, the responses of 30 to 33 out of 100 study participants can be attributed to the placebo effect, the power of the mind to heal.

Science journalist Jo Marchant has written extensively about the mind-body connection and the healing power of the mind. Though initially a skeptic on the subject of placebos, Marchant cites in *Cure* the case of an 11-year-old girl with lupus, a life-threatening, autoimmune condition. Initially the girl was treated with steroids that caused her to lose her hair and gain weight. In addition, her pediatrician used biofeedback and hypnosis to help her cope with stress. Sadly, after two years, the patient's condition deteriorated. When her heart and other organs began to fail, the doctors put her on Cytoxan, a toxic drug with side effects almost as dangerous as the disease itself.

Desperate to find a cure for her child, the girl's mother, a psychologist, shared an academic paper with her daughter's pediatrician, written by psychologist Robert Ader, founder of the field of psychoneuroimmunology, which studies the effect of the mind on health and resistance to disease. Dr. Ader had successfully trained a group of mice to associate Cytoxan with a saccharin solution. He continued to administer the sweetened water, along with half the usual dose of the harsh drug. Remarkably, the mice given the sweetened water lived as long as those treated with the full dose of Cytoxan.

After an extensive review by the ethical board of the hospital where the girl in Dr. Marchant's book was being treated, Bob Ader was permitted to do an experiment. He designed a treatment for the girl using cod liver oil as the alternate substance along with a rose scent to mitigate the fishy taste and smell. He cut the dose of the harsh drug in half and complemented it with the placebo. Within a year, the girl's condition had stabilized and ultimately improved.

GENERAL ONLINE REFERENCES

1. http://www.aging.com/

2. AARP - https://www.aarp.org

3. Retired Brains:
   - https://www.retiredbrains.com

4. Elder One-Stop
   - http://www.elder-one-stop.com

5. Local libraries

6. 3rd Act Magazine
   - https://www.3rdactmagazine.com

7. Suddenly Senior
   - https://www.suddenlysenior.com

8. Community Centers

9. Local Colleges - Continuing Education Classes, sometimes specifically for 50 or 60+

10. Google, Google, Google! (or any search engine) - (and many local libraries have programs to

help you with computer skills if you aren't sure how to go about it)

11. Great Senior Living
    - https://www.greatseniorliving.com

12. TED Talks on Aging

13. https://www.ted.com/topics/aging

14. National Council on Aging - Aging Mastery Program - https://www.ncoa.org/healthy-aging/aging-mastery-program/

15. Next Avenue - https://www.nextavenue.org

16. 60+Me online community for women over 60 http://sixtyandme.com/start/

RECOMMENDED READING

1. Chopra, Deepak. *Ageless Body, Timeless Mind: The Quantum Alternative To Growing Old.* New York: Random House, 2010.

2. Langer, Elinor J. *Counterclockwise: Mindful Health and the Power of Possibility.* New York: Random House, 2009.

3. Magnusson, Margareta. *The Gentle Art of Swedish Death Cleaning: How To Free Yourself and Your Family from a Lifetime of Clutter.* New York: Simon & Schuster, 2010.

4. Leland, John. *Happiness Is a Choice You Make.* New York: Sarah Crichton Books, 2018.

5. Marchant, Jo. *Cure: A Journey into the Science of Mind Over Body.* New York: Random House, 2016.

6. Moore, Thomas. *Ageless Soul: The Lifelong Journey Toward Meaning and Joy.* New York: St. Martin's Press, 2017.

7. Richmond, Lewis. *Aging as a Spiritual Practice: A Contemplative Guide to Growing Old.* New York: Penguin Group, 2012.

8. Robbins, John. *Healthy at 100: The Scientifically Proven Secrets of the World's Healthiest and Longest Living People.* New York: Random House, 2006.

9. Schachter-Shalomi, Zalman and Miller, Ronald S. *From Age-ing to Sage-ing: A Revolutionary Approach to Growing Older.* New York: Grand Central Publishing, 1995.

ABOUT THE AUTHOR

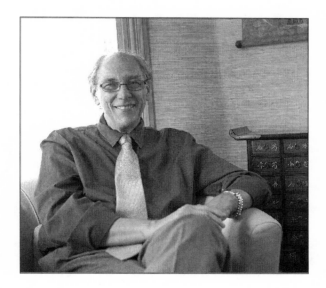

Jason Elias has had a lifelong passion for healing. His earliest memories include watching his Greek Jewish grandmother concoct herbal remedies and poultices in the kitchen of his boyhood home in Brooklyn. He would emulate his beloved elder by "healing" his family and neighbors with grass cuttings and sugar.

As a young man, he studied psychology, acupuncture, and both Chinese and Western Herbal Medicine. His passion led him to study with many master teachers in New York City, California, the Philippines, Japan, China, India, and England. He has been in private practice for more than 40 years, working with clients of all ages. He is the author of four previous books:

- *Feminine Healing: A Woman's Guide to a Healthy Body, Mind, and Spirit* (Warner Books)

- **Chinese Medicine for Maximum Immunity: Understanding the Five Elemental Types for Health and Well-Being** (Three Rivers Press)

- *The A to Z Guide to Healing Herbal Remedies* (Dell Books)

- *Kissing Joy As It Flies: A Journey in Search of Healing and Wholeness* (Five Element Healing Press)

For more information about his work, contact: http://www.fiveelementhealing.net

Made in United States
Orlando, FL
29 July 2022

20296118R00155